SMART WAYS TO STAY YOUNG AND HEALTHY

T0151058

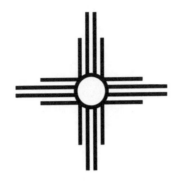

SMART WAYS TO STAY YOUNG AND HEALTHY

BRADLEY GASCOIGNE, M.D.
JULIE IRWIN

RONIN PUBLISHING, INC.

Published by
Ronin Publishing, Inc.
Post Office Box 1035
Berkeley, California 94701

Smart Ways to Stay Young & Healthy
ISBN: 0-914171-49-6

Printed in the United States of America
First printing 1992

9 8 7 6 5 4

Project Editors: Sebastian Orfali and Beverly Potter
Manuscript Editor: Aiden Kelley
Preliminary Editing: Lori Michalos
Proofreader: Ginger Ashworth
Cover Design: Brian Groppe
Illustrations: Roger Margulies, Jean Anderson
Page Composition: Roger Margulies & Don Margulies
Typographic Output: Generic Typography

U.S. Library of Congress Cataloging in Publication Data
Bradley Gascoigne, M.D., & Julie N. Irwin
       Smart Ways to Stay Young & Healthy
              1. Health. 2. Medicine.
       I. Title.

This book is a survey of methods used to promote personal
health. *It does not replace supervision under the skill and
experience of a physician.* Examples given in this book
should be considered general and theoretical. No two
people are alike. The publisher and the author are not responsible for the specific application of this material.
Readers are urged to find a personal physician to help
guide them to better health.

DEDICATION

To Robert L. Cella, M.D., first physician-in-chief at the Kaiser Permanente Medical Center in Martinez, California for his leadership and sense of humor, to

Jim, Jimmy, and Chris for their encouragement and understanding, and

Carol Butterfield, publicist, whose encouragement and guidance in this book's early stages helped it become a reality.

ACKNOWLEDGMENTS

We have gained ideas and insights from many friends, patients, and colleagues. The people listed below have helped most directly, and to them we are indeed grateful. We also express thanks to any others who have also helped us.

Mary Abell, M.D., family practitioner; **Mike Allerton, M.S.**, AIDS educator; **Myrna Allums, R.N., M.S.**, health educator; **Hank Anderson**, minister; **Jean Anderson**, stretching illustrator; **Ginger Ashworth**, editor; **Steve Baker, M.D.**, dermatologist; **Cynthia Bearer, M.D.**, environmental researcher; **Jill Bernstein**, publicist; **Charlene Brooks, Sr. L.V.N.**, clinic nurse; **Carol Butterfield**, publicist; **Alan Chasnoff, M.D.**, ophthalmologist; **Kate Christensen, M.D.**, medical ethicist; **Judith Epstein**, attorney; **Rae Evans, M.D.**, health-care administrator; **Eric Feldman, M.D.**, oncologist; **Gloria Frankl, M.D.**, radiologist; **Brian Groppe**, cover design; **Ann Grove**, physical therapist; **James Harris, D.V.M.**, veterinarian; **Stuart Harrison**, enologist; **Bahman Hayati, M.D.**, physician; **Chuck Hearey, M.D.**, physician; **Ira at Cody's**, book buyer; **Mardy Ireland, Ph.D.**, psychologist; **John Igo, M.D.**, surgeon; **Jim Irwin**, aerobics consultant; **Nate Kaufman, D.D.S.**, dentist; **Harvey Kaymen, M.D.**, health educator; **Aiden Kelley**, editor; **Laura Keranen, M.P.H.**, health educator; **Tupper Kinder**, consultant; **David Lawrence, CEO**, Kaiser Permanente Medical Care Program; **Carol Lundgren**, educator; **Lori Louise Michalos**, editor; **Daniel Margulies & Roger Margulies**, Conquest Designs, Inc. (graphics); **George Matula, M.D.**, AIDS consultant; **Michael Miller, M.D.**, allergist; **Carla Omar**, transcriptionist; **Walt Orenstein, M.D.**, Centers for Disease Control Division Chief; **Sebastian Orfali**, publisher; **Albert Palitz, M.D.**, internist; **Wayne Phillips**, jogging consultant; **Beverly Potter, Ph.D.**, publisher; **Len Pytel**, geriatric consultant; **Rich Rabens, M.D.**, physician; **Herb Rheingruber, M.D.**, obstetrician/gynecologist; **David Ross, Ph.D.**, psychologist; **Dean Ross**, health enthusiast; **Doug Ross, D.C.**, chiropractor; **Bart Rubin, Ph.D.**, psychologist; **Aaron Sanders, Ph.D.**, physicist; **David Sobel, M.D., M.P.H.**, author/health educator; **Becky Tucker**, nutritionist; **Phyllis Ward**, logotherapist; **Tim Weaver**, mountaineer; **Walt Williams, M.D.**, Centers for Disease Control section chief; **Michael Wood**, attorney; **William Wright, M.D.**, psychiatrist.

INTRODUCTION

At a high school reunion a year and a half ago, we first envisioned this book. Our intent ever since has been to write a health book for American adults that is concise, up-to-date, and practical.

Americans are living longer than ever, but how many of those years following retirement are active and independent? One of our goals has been to provide health information to enable us all to live our later years more enjoyably, healthfully, and independently. The knowledge and the technology exist to do so.

In part, this book has been influenced by "Healthy People 2000," the U.S. Department of Health and Human Services' report on health goals for us all for the 1990s. It is clear that each of us can choose a lifestyle that will promote our own good health. In part our book comes from a 450-page U.S. Preventive Task Force report that critically looked at 169 medical practices in traditional Western medicine and asked, "What is the evidence to continue such practices?" In part it was inspired by *50 Simple Things You Can Do to Save the Earth*, which reminds us that people like concise books. And this book springs from our own personal readings. These "favorite readings" are included at the end of each chapter.

Our book has also been influenced by mentors such as Dr. Edward Mortimer, currently at Case Western Reserve Medical Center, who admonished his residents with that acronym, K.I.S.S. (Keep It Simple Stupid). And by Dr. Mary Abell of Tulane Medical Center who continues to emphasize the value of prevention in our lives, and the need for health research concerning women as well as men. We were also influenced by Dr. Robert Cella, former head physician at one of the Kaiser Permanente Hospitals in Northern California, who preached the value of one-page memos. And finally we are indebted to writers and leaders such as Dr. David Lawrence, Harold Kushner, Dr. David Sobel, Laura Keranen, Dolores Curran, John-Henry Pfifferling, and Norman Cousins whose writings and counseling have inspired many.

We have a tremendously unrealized health potential in this country. It is sobering to realize that our U.S. estimated life span of 75 years trails that of Japan by nearly 5 years. The proportion of Americans over 65 is growing, and will have doubled by early next century. Living longer isn't always better, but it's nice to have the option.

Smart Ways to Stay Young and Healthy is intended to help keep your life and later years healthy and independent.

Julie Irwin
Bradley Gascoigne, M.D.
December 1991

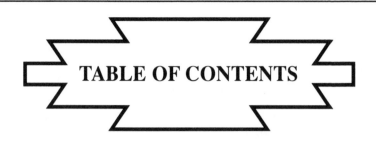

TABLE OF CONTENTS

I. Activities for Your Body

II. Smart Nutrition

III. Preventive Steps

IV. Risks to Avoid

V. Emotional Well-Being

FIVE WORTHWHILE
HEALTH PUBLICATIONS

Berkeley Wellness Letter, University of California, Subscription Dept., P.O. Box 420148, Palm Coast, FL 32142

Harvard Health Letter, Subscription Dept., P.O. Box 420299, Palm Coast, FL 32142-9858

John Hopkins Medical Letter, *Health after 50*, Subscription Dept. Box 420179, Palm Coast, FL 32142

Mayo Clinic Health Letter, Mayo Clinic, 200 1st St. S.W., Rochester, MN 55905

Prevention® magazine, c/o Rodale Press, 33 East Minor Street, Emmaus, PA 18098

Each is issued monthly.

SMART WAYS TO STAY YOUNG AND HEALTHY

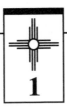

1

EXERCISE AEROBICALLY

As a friend recently put it, "If I exercise regularly, everything else takes care of itself." He went on to say that when he exercises, he sleeps better, he tends to eat better, he has more energy, he is less apt to smoke, and he generally feels less stressed. There's a lot of truth in what he says.

Heart disease kills more than 700,000 people each year in this country, more than cancer or any other disease. A major factor in these deaths is lack of exercise. Lack of exercise is present in these people *twice as often* as any other cardiac risk factor that can be changed by a person's behavior.

Benefits of Aerobic Exercise

Aerobic exercise is exercise which is continuous, and which utilizes your muscles, increases your heart rate, and lasts for a minimum of twelve minutes.

The benefits of aerobics are many and varied. Here are some taken from the Department of Health and Human Services report *Healthy People 2000*, from a medical study of the benefits of jogging, and from our own personal experiences:
- Reduces risk of heart disease
- Allows easier maintenance of normal weight
- Lowers blood pressure
- Reduces discomfort from PMS (Premenstrual Syndrome)
- Increases bone strength and density
- Reduces chance of depression or anxiety
- Reduces frequency and severity of lower back pain
- Allows longer maintenance of independent living among the elderly
- Reduces smoking
- Gives better immunity to colds and minor infections
- Allows better management of diabetes and may even *prevent* diabetes

- Decreases levels of blood cholesterol and lipids
- Lowers rates of colon and breast cancer
- Lowers risk of stroke
- Increases flexibility
- Develops firmer muscles
- Gives greater endurance
- Allows sounder sleep
- Promotes greater self-esteem
- Increases life expectancy.

Drawbacks to Aerobic Exercise

Aerobic programs do increase your chance of injuries, usually to the ankles, knees, or hips. To lessen your chance of injuries, be sure to stretch regularly, use good equipment (especially shoes), and build up your program *gradually*! Before you embark on a vigorous exercise program, discuss your own medical status with your health-care provider.

Aerobic Choices

Those available today range from lap swimming, water calisthenics, bicycling, jazzercise, indoor treadmills, and jogging to in-line skating, fast walking, mall walking, cross-country skiing, StairMaster®, and triathlons. The key is to find one, or more, that are interesting to you.

How Much Exercise?

How much exercise per session, how many sessions a week, is the right balance between the benefits of aerobic exercise and the risk of injuries from overdoing it? And how much will you keep up with, given your lifestyle and present commitments? We probably all know people who started swimming laps, for example, six days a week, and kept it up for months or even years, and then quit. They burned out, got injured, lost interest, or whatever. How much swimming or other aerobic exercise can you keep up *for your lifetime*?

Answers to these questions depend on to whom you talk. There is no absolute answer that fits everyone. Dr. Ken Cooper, author of *Aerobics,* and president and founder of the Aerobics Center in Dallas, Texas, says that "anyone who runs more than fifteen miles per week is doing so for other than health reasons." Some recommend five to ten miles a week of jogging, for example, as a lower limit to aim for, with fifteen miles a week as an upper limit. Most emphasize duration rather than distance. It's generally agreed that 20–30 minutes per session, with three or four sessions each week, is of the greatest long-term benefit. *Moderation* is the key.

When to Exercise?

1. First thing in the morning if you're a procrastinator.
2. In the middle of the morning, if that's when you can coordinate your schedule with a friend or an aerobics class or another group.
3. At lunch hour, if you exercise to reduce work-related stress.
4. Late in the afternoon (before dinner), if you want to maximize the weight-losing benefits of aerobic exercise.
5. At the end of your workday, if you want to let the rush-hour commute thin out before driving home.
6. Anytime during the day, but not less than 3 or 4 hours before bedtime, if you want to sleep better at night.

Recommendations

1. Start a *moderate* aerobic exercise program that you can include three times in your weekly schedule for 20 minutes each session. Include extra time for stretching. Gradually increase to four 30-minute sessions per week.
2. Wherever possible, walk short distances instead of driving or riding.
3. Whenever possible, walk up a flight of stairs instead of taking an elevator.

Favorite Reading

Fit or Fat, by Covert Bailey. Boston, MA: Houghton Mifflin, 1977, 120 pgs.

Answer:

In-water exercise classes

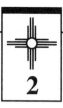

2

TAKE A POWER NAP

Sleep experts now say that more than half of Americans are sleep deprived, and that most of us are getting sixty to ninety minutes *less* sleep than we need. Are you cheating yourself on sleep?

Why Are Naps Important?

Everybody is different, but young and middle-aged adults usually need seven to nine hours of sleep each night in order to feel honestly rested. Older adults may actually need less, which can be a surprise. Knowing how much sleep is best for you takes experimenting. If you can't easily get this much sleep because of children or busy schedules, learn the art of a power nap.

In his book *What They Still Don't Teach You at Harvard Business School*, Clevelander Mark McCormack describes how he blocks out time in his afternoon schedule for a nap. His secretary knows that this time is to be guarded just as other important commitments would be.

Dr. Tom Plaut, national asthma expert from Amherst, Massachusetts, and author of *Children with Asthma*, recently said while traveling, "Give me five minutes for a nap," between dropping off his luggage and heading out to dinner. He explained how he learned the art of cat napping to get through internship and residency. Now he uses it daily.

We live in a society in which getting by with less sleep than we need is considered by some to be macho, partly because of our Puritan work ethic. However, the toll on our personal health, as well as our personalities, is considerable. Cultures in which a

What percent of Americans say they took a nap in the past 24 hours?

siesta is still commonplace may know something about optimal functioning that we've lost sight of. In fact, a recent study by NASA and Professor Dinges of the University of Pennsylvania showed that pilots who were relieved for a 20-minute-plus nap in flight carried out later tasks significantly better.

For many people, 20 minutes at a time works best. If you sleep longer than 35 or 40 minutes during the day, it can leave you feeling more sluggish than rested. Perhaps this fact is why TM (transcendental meditation) sessions traditionally last 20 minutes. The greatest benefit is derived by naps during the "siesta zone" (noon to 4 p.m.).

Recommendation

Learn the art of a power nap. Lock your office door, or find a quiet room. Unplug your phone. Use a couch, a futon, or even the floor. Keep a pillow in your filing cabinet. Discover what length of nap or relaxation in the middle of the day works best for you.

Favorite Reading

You Don't Have to Go Home from Work Exhausted, by Ann McGee-Cooper, Duane Trammell, and Barbara Lau. Dallas, TX: Bowin & Rogers, 1990, 349 pgs.

3

STRETCH EACH MORNING

Why Stretching Is Important

Stretching is a relaxed, sustained extension of a specific muscle, without bouncing, intended to promote tissue relaxation in a non-competitive manner. There are many advantages to stretching every day, whether you are already physically fit or struggling to get there. Some people say that stretching in the morning puts them more in touch with their bodies. Others claim that it simply helps them to wake up. Some claim it improves their circulation or improves their posture. Others use stretching to increase flexibility and to reduce muscle tightness. Some stretch to avoid exercise-induced injuries. And for many others, stretching in the morning gives them a greater zest for life.

Recommendation

Develop your own morning stretching routine according to your likes and needs. Take into account any past injuries. Since low back pain, ankle injuries, poor posture, and tight neck muscles are so common in our society, we've included several stretches especially for these areas. What follows are descriptions and illustrations of our ten favorite morning exercises and stretches. These can easily be done in five to ten minutes before moving on to the rest of your day. Since these are all non-impact exercises, pregnant women can safely perform them well into their third trimester, as long as they don't have a history of premature labor. Remember not to bounce, but to stretch slowly, for 20 to 30 seconds for each stretch. Be gentle, and don't stretch to the point of pain.

How many separate muscles are there in the human body?

Stretching Exercises

1. Double knees to chest

This exercise is intended to loosen up your lower back. While lying on the floor (or even while still in bed) and on your back, raise both knees gradually to your chest, clasp your hands around the fronts of your knees, and hold for 30 seconds as you feel a gentle stretch in your lower back.

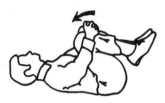

2. Single knee to chest

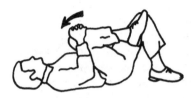

Here is another exercise to loosen up your lower back. While still on your back, with one leg extended, clasp one knee with your hands to your chest. Release, straighten that leg, and clasp the opposite knee to your chest. Do each movement 10 to 20 times.

3. Abdominal curls

This exercise will strengthen your abdominal muscles, and protect your back as a result. Still on your back, with your knees flexed half-way, place each hand on the opposite shoulder. Bend your trunk until your shoulderblades are off the ground. Relax. Repeat 10 to 20 times.

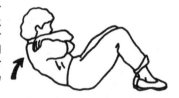

4. Press-ups or push-ups

These exercises can be done to either extend and stretch your trunk, or to strengthen your upper chest and pectoralis muscles. From a position lying on your stomach, raise your head, shoulders, and upper body off the ground, leaving your hips and lower body still on the floor (press-ups) or pushing your entire body off the floor (push-ups). Repeat 5 to 25 times.

5. Superman lifts

These exercises will strengthen the paraspinal muscles, which run the length of your back. While on your abdomen, extend both your arms and your legs. Next, raise your left arm and your left leg slightly. As you lower these, raise the opposite arm and leg. Alternate lifts and repeat for 20 to 60 seconds.

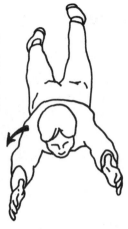

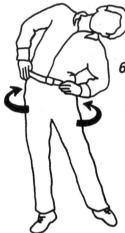

6. Around the world

To loosen the muscles of your abdomen and sides, stand with your hands on your hips and your knees bent slightly (not locked). Concentrate on keeping your abdominal and buttock muscles tight for pelvic stabilization. Arch backward at the waist and hold for 3 to 5 seconds. Slowly lean to one side and feel a gentle stretch in your opposite side above the waist. Continue around until your head is in front of your knees. Hold briefly, then continue around to your other side and then backward. Complete 5 to 10 rotations in each direction.

7. Neck extensions

This stretch is intended to counteract the hunched-back posture some of us develop from sitting at desks or computers all day. Sit comfortably. With up-right posture, clasp your hands behind your head, with your elbows approximately 45 degrees out to the sides. Slowly arch your neck backward until you can see the ceiling (imagine a string lifting your breastbone upwards). Keep your elbows back. Hold for 15 seconds. Relax and repeat.

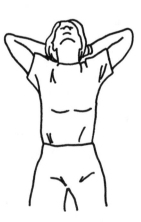

8. Neck and trunk rotations

This exercise will loosen the rotational muscles of your neck and upper trunk. While sitting upright with your lower back arched and your chin level, interlock your fingers (curled) several inches in front of your chin. Slowly rotate your arms, trunk, head, and neck about 90 degrees to one side. Pause briefly. Rotate 180 degrees back to the opposite side. Repeat to each side 10 to 20 times.

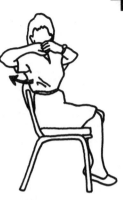

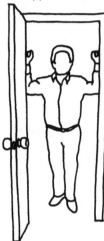

9. Doorway shoulder extensions

This exercise will broaden and relax the chest and anterior shoulder muscles. Stand in a doorway with one foot about 12 inches behind the other and outside of the doorway. Grasp the door frame with each hand raised, so that your elbows are bent 90 degrees and level with your shoulders. Lean forward slowly to extend your shoulders backward with the stretch in your upper chest. Hold for 15 seconds. Switch feet position and repeat stretch for another 15 seconds.

10. Ankle inversions

This stretch is intended to increase the strength and the flexibility of your lateral (outer) ankles, and is especially helpful if you tend to suffer ankle sprains. Allow only a slight stretch initially until you build up the strength in this part of your body. Stand, holding onto a chair or table for balance, and turn in (invert) one ankle until you feel a slight stretch in the outer portion just beneath your heel bone. Hold for 10 to 30 seconds. Repeat with the opposite ankle slowly turned inward.

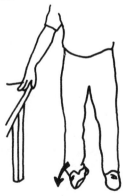

Stretching
illustrations by
Jean Anderson

Favorite Reading

Stretching, by Bob Anderson, illustrated by Jean Anderson. Bolinas, CA: Shelter Publication, 1980, 192 pgs.

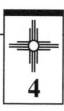

4

TAKE GOOD CARE OF YOUR BACK

These days you can get an artificial knee if you need one, or an artificial hip. You can even get a new liver, a new kidney, or a heart-lung transplant. But as of now you get only one back, and it needs to last your lifetime. Some people can be helped with back surgery, such as fusing together two or more vertebrae, but it's not the same as getting a new back.

How Common Are Back Problems?

- 100 million people in this country suffer back pain each year.
- 80 to 90% of Americans will be affected at some time in their lives by back trouble.
- Surgery for ruptured discs is performed more than 100,000 times each year, at an average cost of $15,000.

Recommendations and Cautions

1. If your car has cruise control, use it when you can; doing so will take some strain off the lower right part of your back.
2. Use lower back stretches in the morning to keep your back flexible (see Chapter 3).
3. Both at home and at work, use chairs that have proper support. The seat shouldn't be too deep (front to back). While sitting, use a low back pillow or orthopedic support such as those sold in medical supply stores or chiropractic and physical-therapy offices.
4. Do bent-knee sit-ups and abdominal curl exercises to strengthen your abdominal muscles, which helps your back.
5. When lifting objects, bend your knees so that the strain is on your thigh muscles rather than your back muscles.
6. Lose weight. Losing one pound of excess weight will take ten pounds of stress off your lower back!
7. Sleep on a firm mattress or a Japanese futon instead of a soft mattress or a waterbed.
8. Sleep on your back or your side, with your legs partially bent, to reduce strain on your back.

How many bones are there in the human spine?

9. If you carry a thick wallet in your back pocket, keep it somewhere else when sitting (this includes driving time).
10. Get yourself and your back in shape during pregnancy and after childbirth. You need to be ready to carry your baby around when he or she is a year old and weighs over 20 pounds.
11. Quit smoking! Smoking can contribute to degeneration of the discs between your vertebrae by reducing their blood supply.
12. If your work requires bending, such as vacuuming or shoveling, bend backward several times at least once every hour.
13. If you work with weights, consult with a trainer. Weightlifting can put a tremendous strain on the lower back. As Jose Canseco of the Oakland A's says, "I weight train. I don't weightlift," when talking about his back conditioning.
14. Exercise aerobically. Brisk walking, swimming, and bicycling are considered the three best aerobic exercises for your back.

Recommended Resources

Video: *Say Good-bye to Back Pain* by the YMCA and Dr. Hans Kraus. Call your local chapter to order it.

Back Support: McCarty's Sacro-Ease®, Coeur d'Alene, ID, 800-635-3557.

Favorite Reading

Treat Your Own Back, by Robin McKenzie. Waikanae, New Zealand: Spinal Publications, 1985, 73 pgs. (Available through Orthopedic Physical Therapy Products, Box 41009, Minneapolis, MN 55441; 800-367-7393.)

The Y's Way to a Healthy Back, by Alexander Melleby. Clinton, NJ: New Win Publishing, 1982, 174 pgs.

Answer:

26 (7 cervical, 12 thoracic, 5 lumbar, the sacrum, and the coccyx or tailbone)

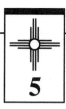

5

BRUSH AND FLOSS YOUR TEETH

"I can tell when I'm stressed in my life, because flossing my teeth is first to go," said author and health educator Dr. David Sobel recently. Many people leave dental care for the time that's left over after everything else is done. That may work . . . until problems arise.

Why Is Tooth Care Important?

Have you ever wondered why you haven't seen pictures of George Washington smiling? Or Thomas Jefferson? Or James Madison? Probably they were not very proud of their smiles or, more specifically, their teeth! Even as recently as a century ago, most people's teeth didn't last their lifetimes. Today, with modern dental expertise and proper care, we can expect to keep our teeth for our entire lives.

Our first permanent teeth erupt at age 5 or 6, and we have most of them by age 20. The average life span of Americans is well over 70, which means keeping our adult teeth for 60 to 80 years. But to keep our teeth that long takes consistent daily attention. We must remove all plaque every day, before it hardens. The bacteria that cause tooth decay and bone loss live in plaque.

How Common Are Dental and Oral Disease?

- 16% of Americans have lost all of their original teeth by the time they are 60 years old.
- 75% of American adults have periodontal (gum) disease, which is the leading cause of tooth loss after age 35.
- Almost 30,000 new cases of oral cancer will be detected this year, resulting in more than 8,000 deaths.
- In 1980, 71% of nine-year-olds had cavities; by 1990 that had dropped to 50%.

What percent of Americans say they have flossed their teeth in the past 24 hours?

Recommendations

Daily brushing and regular dental checkups are the cornerstones of proper dental care. In addition:
1. Floss your teeth every day.
2. If you have difficulty holding dental floss with your fingers, buy a 99-cent Y-shaped flossing fork.
3. Take advantage of fluoride, which strengthens your teeth against decay. Daily use of fluoride mouthrinse is helpful for adults as well as children.
4. Buy "disclosing tablets" at a drug store, and chew one occasionally after brushing; it will stain any plaque that's left on your teeth. Change your brushing technique to reach spots you've been missing.
5. Make sure your dentist screens for signs of oral cancer during your regular dental exams.
6. In between visits to your dentist, use a mirror to check your own lips, gums, and cheeks for sores or color changes.
7. If you lose a tooth in an accident, thoroughly rinse the tooth off, reinsert it promptly, and see your dentist immediately. If you can't reinsert the tooth, transport it in milk.
8. Chew sugarless rather than sugared gum.
9. Don't chew tobacco.

Recommended Resource

For more thorough plaque removal, in addition to flossing, use Interplak® toothbrushes, c/o Bausch and Lomb, Oral Care Division, Georgia (800-334-4031).

Favorite Reading

New Dimensions, edited by Jill Hightower, 4863 Fredericksburg Rd., San Antonio, TX 78229, a quarterly newsletter.

Answer:
25%

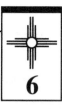

6

BREATHE FOR RELAXATION

In 1984 appeared the book *Peak Performance: Mental Training Techniques of the World's Greatest Athletes* by sports psychologist Charles Garfield, revealing the training secrets of the then-dominant Soviet and East German Olympic athletes. The author tells how he used their methods of relaxation and visualization to weightlift 365 lbs., even though he hadn't seriously weight trained for eight years, and this had been his previous "personal best." Among the various techniques he employed, relaxation breathing is probably the easiest to learn for yourself. Learn the following technique as a means to relax.

Technique

Find a quiet room. Seat yourself so that you are fully upright. Rest your arms comfortably on your thighs. As you relax, you may choose to close your eyes. Take in a slow, full breath through your nose, fully using first your abdominal and then your chest muscles. Hold your breath for a few seconds. Exhale through your mouth. As you breathe out, feel the weight and tension drain from your shoulders, your neck, and the rest of your body.

Repeat the above sequence for 10 to 15 minutes a day until it becomes automatic. This technique easily leads into other relaxation techniques, such as visualizing the blood flowing into your arms and hands as you relax your arms and feel the warmth reach the tips of your fingers. It can be used as a part of a 20-minute period of relaxation and meditation to recharge yourself in the middle of the day. Or it can be used as a trial visualization of an upcoming performance or athletic feat. For all of these, relaxed breathing, from one long breath to a twenty-minute session, will help.

Approximately how many quarts of air does the average adult breathe in and out every day?

Recommendations

1. Practice the above breathing relaxation sequence for 10 to 15 minutes daily until it becomes second nature.
2. As an example of when to use breathing for relaxation, when you hear the first ring of your telephone, take a long relaxing breath before picking up the receiver.
3. When you must answer a difficult question, take a long breath, and breathe out your tension and anxiety as you speak.

Favorite Reading

The Relaxation and Stress Reduction Workbook by Martha Davis, Ph.D., Elizabeth Robbins Eshelman, M.S.W., and Mathew McKay, Ph.D. Oakland, CA: New Harbinger Publications, 3d edition, 1988, 249 pgs. Winner of the 1982 Medical Self-Care Book Award.

7

DO THESE FOR YOUR BODY ALSO

1. If you spend considerable amounts of time in bright sunshine, you can decrease the risk of cataracts by wearing sunglasses that filter more than 50% of UVA and UVB rays.
2. If you suffer from arthritis, read *The Arthritis Help Book*, by Kate Lorig, R.N., Ph.D., and James Fries, M.D. Reading, PA: Addison-Wesley, 1990.
3. If you're over 40, get your eyes screened for glaucoma; the test is quick and painless.
4. If you suffer from canker sores in your mouth, apply tincture of iodine with a cotton-tipped swab to the sores to dry them up more quickly.
5. To lessen the severity of an early cold, fill a bowl with boiling water, use a towel to make a tent over your head above the bowl, and breathe in the warm water vapor through your nostrils.
6. If you have difficulties with dribbling or urinary incontinence, discuss the subject with your doctor. Many cases are treatable, but only half the adults with this embarrassing condition discuss it with their health-care provider.
7. "If you are depressed, take up gardening; working with the soil is therapeutic." Dr. Sherman, 19th-century Columbus, Ohio, general practitioner.
8. For those who suffer from seasonal affective disorder (S.A.D., "winter depression"), investigate Medic-Light's ultraviolet-free indoor lights (800-LIGHT-25) to lessen your winter doldrums.
9. Listen to your body so as to detect injuries or oncoming illnesses in their early stages.

Favorite Reading

365 Health Hints, by Don Powell. New York: Simon & Schuster, 1990, 372 pgs.

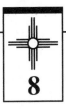

8

KEEP YOUR BONES
YOUNG AND HEALTHY

After the age of 30 to 35, we actually begin losing bone mass. This may not have been as important a century ago, when Americans had a much shorter life expectancy. But today this thinning of our bones, known as osteoporosis, is definitely a problem. The most common results of osteoporosis are broken hips, wrist fractures, compression fractures of our spine's vertebrae, and a hunched-back posture. We can actually become shorter as we age. And women, especially women after menopause, are the ones most vulnerable to this process.

How Common Are Osteoporosis and
Related Bone Fractures?

- More than 20 million adults in the U.S. have osteoporosis.
- There are more than 500,000 episodes of vertebral fractures each year resulting from this condition.
- Every year, more than 250,000 people break their hip; among those, more than 20,000 die within six months from the complications.
- 40% of women will suffer at least one spinal fracture by age 80.

Who Is Most at Risk for Osteoporosis?

According to Dr. David Fardon's *Osteoporosis* and several other recent scientific reports, risk factors for osteoporosis can differ greatly for different demographic groups, as shown in the table here.

Relative Risk of Osteoporosis

High Risk	Low Risk
Females	Males
Caucasians and Orientals	Blacks
Family history of osteoporosis	No family history of osteoporosis
Northern European heritage	Mediterranean heritage
Surgical menopause	Normal menopause
Early menopause	Late menopause
Limited exercise	Regular, lifelong exercise
Calcium-poor diet	Calcium-rich diet
Smoking	Nonsmoking
Regular alcohol intake	Nondrinker
Fair skin	Dark skin
Red or blond hair	Dark hair
Loose, clear, wrinkled skin	Tough, thick skin
Loose joints and muscles	Tight joints
Flat feet	Sturdy arches
Scoliosis	No scoliosis
Small muscles	Large muscles
Being underweight	Being overweight
Periodontal disease	Healthy teeth and gums
Illness causing inactivity	High level of activity
Stomach and bowel disease	Normal stomach
Medicines that weaken bone (such as anti-seizure medications)	No medicine intake
Previous fractures	No fractures
Loss of height	No loss of height
Rheumatoid arthritis	Definite osteoarthritis
Anorexia nervosa	Normal weight
Subtle excess of thyroid hormone medication	Appropriate thyroid drug level

If you have three or more of the factors in the left-hand column, you are at significant risk for osteoporosis.

Adapted from *Osteoporosis* by Dr. David Fardon.

Recommendations

1. Be physically active both while young *and* during your later years.
2. Get enough calcium in your diet; see the following table. Children and adults need 800 mg. a day. Adolescents, pregnant women, breast-feeding mothers, and women over 55 require 1000–1500 mg. per day.
3. Include 400 units of vitamin D, which is necessary for healthy bone formation, in your daily diet.
4. For women at or past menopause, consider daily estrogen supplements. (Before starting on such a daily regimen, discuss the risks and benefits with your gynecologist or nurse practitioner.)
5. Find out about the newly proven drug etidronate (Didronil®).
6. Drink fluoridated water. Population studies in the U. S., England, and Finland show fewer hip fractures in those groups who do. Check with your local water district to find out whether or not your water is fluoridated.

Elemental Calcium Content

Calcium source	Single serving	Amount of Calcium
Milk (skim or whole)	8 oz. glass	300 mg.
Cheese	1 oz.	240 mg.
Pudding	1 cup	300 mg.
Yogurt	6 oz.	300 mg.
Spinach (cooked)	4 oz. (1/2 cup)	125 mg.
Broccoli (cooked)	4 oz. (1/2 cup)	100 mg.
Collard Greens (cooked)	4 oz. (1/2 cup)	75 mg.
Tofu (cooked)	2 oz.	50 mg.
Bony Fish (canned)	4 oz.	250 mg.
Almonds	2 oz.	150 mg.
Calcium Supplements	1 Tablet	100–500 mg.
Tums® Antacids	1 Tablet	200–300 mg.
Rolaids® (sodium-free)	1 Tablet	220 mg.

Adapted from National Dairy Board data.

Word of caution: Extra calcium may be a problem for those prone to kidney stones.

Recommended Resource

For more information contact The National Osteoporosis Foundation, 2100 M St. NW, Suite 602, Washington, DC 20037; 202-223-2226.

Favorite Reading

Osteoporosis, by David Fardon, M.D. Tucson, AZ: The Body Press, 1985, 276 pgs.

Answer:
206 bones

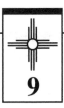

9

EAT FIVE FRUITS
OR VEGETABLES A DAY

Nutritional advice used to be fairly straightforward: eat three square meals a day and get the recommended daily amounts (RDAs) of vitamins and minerals. There were the four basic food groups (dairy, meats, fruits and vegetables, and breads and cereals), and you were supposed to reasonably divide your intake among them. But with high rates in this country of strokes, elevated blood pressures, and heart attacks, concern has arisen about our diets, which are often high in animal fat, overly salted, preservative-laden, artificially colored, and increasingly processed. Health experts believe 33 to 35% of cancers are affected by our diets. As nutritional expert Edward Blonz, Ph.D., recently wrote, "We now know that a good diet means much more than preventing a deficiency."

USDA Dietary Guidelines

In 1980 the official nutritional guidelines put out by the U.S. Department of Agriculture were revised to read as follows.

1. Eat a variety of foods.
2. Maintain ideal body fat.
3. Avoid excessive saturated fat, and cholesterol.
4. Avoid excessive sodium and salt.
5. Avoid excessive sugar.
6. Eat foods with starch and fiber.
7. Drink only moderate amounts of alcohol.

These still remain wise advice, but need to be supplemented in light of more recent information. To show how far nutritional thinking has changed, in the spring of 1991 the Physician's Committee for Responsible Medicine proposed replacing the traditional four food groups with a new four: vegetables, grains, legumes, and fruits.

Recommendations

1. At least once a week, have legumes as your main source of protein; legumes include lima beans, kidney beans, navy beans, pinto beans, soybeans, peanuts (and peanut butter), lentils, split peas, black-eyed peas, and chickpeas.
2. Include complex carbohydrates (whole grains, pastas, breads, cereals, and potatoes) in your diet; avoid simple sugar.
3. Include a daily source of fiber (see Chapter 11).
4. Cut back on fat, especially animal fat and saturated fats. Omega-3 oils found in salmon, tuna, sardines, and mackerel probably protect us from heart disease, but animal fats, which are found in meats and dairy products, increase our risk of heart disease.
5. Get enough iron (found in lean meats, beans, fish, whole-grain products, and iron-enriched cereals), which is important in red-blood-cell formation and is especially important for children and menstruating women.
6. Avoid salt and too much sodium if you have high blood pressure and are salt sensitive; check with your physician.
7. Consider Tabasco® sauce as a substitute for salt.
8. Include at least 800 mg. of calcium in your daily diet (see Chapter 8).
9. Eat regular breakfasts, which enhance morning performance.
10. Avoid large dinners, which put on extra weight.
11. Include daily sources of Vitamin A, which contains beta carotene and which is considered protective against cancer, and is found in carrots, sweet potatoes, peaches, apricots, cantaloupes, spinach, squash, and papaya.
12. Avoid the cancer-causing substances that may be produced by frying, broiling, or barbecuing chicken, meat, and fish; instead, try to microwave, stew, boil, or poach meats you eat.
13. Limit caffeine intake to less than four cups of coffee per day.
14. Probably the soundest and simplest dietary advice these days is: *include five servings of fruits or vegetables in your daily diet . . .* and you will avoid many of the health risks mentioned above.

Favorite Reading

The gold standard of nutrition books remains *Jane Brody's Nutrition Book.* New York: Bantam Books, 1981, 553 pgs.

Answer:

Celery, carrots, tomatoes, beets, lettuce, spinach, parsley, and watercress

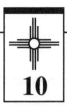

10

KEEP YOUR CHOLESTEROL BELOW 200

Why is the subject of cholesterol so confusing? It's no wonder, with doctors speaking of cholesterol, triglycerides, saturated fats, unsaturated fats, heavy-density lipoproteins, low-density lipoproteins, HDLs vs. LDLs, "good fats" vs. "bad fats," and fasting vs. non-fasting results. To simplify the subject, remember that, in general, the lower your blood cholesterol is, the better. With less fat circulating in your bloodstream, less gets deposited over time on the inner lining of the coronary blood vessels supplying your heart. If the fat deposits (plaques) get too large, a heart attack occurs. Americans suffer 1,500,000 heart attacks and 500,000 deaths every year from this disease.

How Much of Your Diet Is Fat?

Do you know what percentage of your regular calories comes from fat? Here's how to figure it out. On almost every food package is a list that breaks down each serving into grams of fat, carbohydrates, calories, and so on.

1. Take the number of grams of fat per serving.
2. Multiply this number by 9 to get the number of calories from fat.
3. Divide this number by the number of calories per serving; this gives the portion of calories that come from fat.

Beware of foods in which more than 35% of the calories come from fat.

Heart disease is responsible for more deaths in this country each year than all types of cancer combined. True or false?

23

Recommendations

1. Get your blood cholesterol measured every five years; a non-fasting test is acceptable. If it is 200 or less, you can relax.
2. If it is more than 200, make two or three dietary changes (see chart at the end of this chapter), exercise more, and get your level retested every 3 to 6 months, as recommended by your health-care provider.
3. Keep your total fat intake to less than 30% of your daily caloric total (the American average is 37%).
4. Keep your cholesterol intake to less than 300 mg. per day.
5. Include foods that are high in soluble fiber (see Chapter 11).
6. Switch from whole milk or lowfat to 1% or skim; you get the same amount of calcium and protein, but fewer calories and less cholesterol.
7. Ask your health-care provider about the benefits of niacin and lovastatin in shrinking fat deposits inside our blood vessels.
8. Use garlic in moderate amounts to help moderate cholesterol levels (Tulane Medical Center research).
9. Cook with oils that are low in saturated fats, and that contain 20% or less saturated fat in the following list:

Canola oil	6%	Soybean oil	15%
Almond oil	8%	Peanut oil	17%
Safflower oil	9%	Wheat germ oil	19%
Walnut oil	9%	Cottonseed oil	26%
Sunflower oil	10%	Palm oil	49%
Corn oil	13%	Cocoa butter oil	59%
Olive oil	14%	Palm kernel oil	81%
Sesame oil	14%	Coconut oil	87%

10. Avoid saturated fats (butter, coconut oil, palm oil, lard or shortening, egg yolks, all animal fat).
11. Get your significant other involved in your cholesterol-control program.
12. Exercise.
13. Don't smoke.
14. Xerox the following tables on how to lower cholesterol (pages 26 and 27) and post it on your refrigerator door.

Favorite Reading

Lean Toward Health, 22-page booklet, free from Henry J. Kaiser Family Foundation in collaboration with The Partners for Better Health, through the National Center for Nutrition and Dietetics, 800-366-1655.

Prevention Magazine's *Guide to Cutting Your Cholesterol.* Emmaus, PA: Rodale Press, 1990, 40 pgs.

EASY Options
for Lowering Cholesterol through Diet

Food Groups	Option

1. Meat	• Reduce current portion size by 1/3;
	   aim for 3–4 oz. serving
	• Have meat 1/2 as often as you usually do;
	   aim for 3–4 times per week
	• Buy leanest cuts & trim visible fat

2. Eggs	• Limit yolks to 3 per week
	• Substitute 2 egg whites for each whole egg
	   in recipes
	• Use egg substitutes (like Egg Beaters®)
	   in cooking

3. Milk & Cheese	• Use low or nonfat instead of whole milk & yogurt • Use nonfat evaporated milk as coffee lightener • Choose part skim cheeses
4. Added Fats: Spreads (butter, margarine, mayo), Cooking Oils, Salad Dressing	• Reduce to 6 tsp. per day • Avoid fats labeled as hydrogenated • Switch from butter to unsaturated margarine
5. Poultry	• Limit portion: 2 small or 1 large piece • Choose light meat • Remove skin
6. Fish	• Eat fish instead of meat or poultry • Use waterpacked (not oil) tuna
7. Fruits & Vegetables	• Eat more of these • Use for snacks & dessert • Have a salad at least once a day
8. Beans, Grains, & Pasta, Including Bread	• Use meatless sauce with pasta • Substitute beans or tofu for meat in casseroles • Have 1 or 2 meatless days a week using beans & grains as main source of protein
9. Sweets	• Choose angel food cake, sherbet
10. Preparation	• Broil, microwave, or barbecue • Use minimal oil for cooking • Chill stews and soups; skim fat off top

AMBITIOUS Options
for Lowering Cholesterol through Diet

Food Groups	Option
1. Meat	• Limit portion size to 3 oz. (size of a deck of cards) • Limit red meat to 1–2 times per week
2. Eggs	• Limit yolks to 2 or fewer per week
3. Milk & Cheese	• Use nonfat milk & yogurt only • Limit cheese to part skim 3 oz. or less per week
4. Added Fats: Spreads (butter, margarine, mayo) Cooking Oils, Salad Dressing	• Use 4 tsp. or less per day • Choose oil-free salad dressings
5. Poultry	• Restrict to skinless light meat, 3 oz., fewer than 4 times a week
6. Fish	• Eat fish as often as desired
7. Fruits & Vegetables	• Unlimited; aim for 4–8 servings per day
8. Beans, Grains, & Pasta, Including Bread	• Unlimited; aim for 4–8 servings per day
9. Sweets	• Eat fresh fruit • Avoid bakery goods & pastries
10. Preparation	• Use nonstick spray or liquid (wine, broth) for stove top cooking

NOTE: Eating oat bran 2–3 times per day in cereals or muffins can lower cholesterol.

POST ON YOUR REFRIGERATOR!

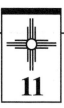

11

TAKE ADVANTAGE OF FIBER

Some experts condense current nutritional advice into the saying, "more fiber, less fat." According to the National Cancer Institute, adult Americans only eat about 11 grams of fiber in their daily diet. The recommended guidelines call for 25 to 40 grams per day.

Benefits of Fiber

Several conditions and diseases are ameliorated by the use of fiber, which contributes to:

1. Decreased incidence of cancer of the colon and rectum
2. Decreased incidence of breast cancer
3. Lowering of blood cholesterol levels (and thereby a decreased risk of coronary artery heart disease)
4. Better control of sugar levels and diabetes
5. Decreased likelihood of diverticulitis (an inflammatory disease of the intestines)
6. Less weight gain
7. Less frequent constipation.

Sources of Fiber

Foods rich in fiber include a variety of whole grains (wheat, rice, oats, corn, and barley) as found in cereals, breads, and muffins. Specific fruits highest in fiber include grapefruits and oranges (with their pulp), bananas, prunes, pears, figs, and apples (with their skins). Vegetable examples would be peas, green beans, lima beans, dried beans, and soybeans. Nuts and various seeds are other sources. A baked potato with its skin contains 4.2 grams of fiber. The following table lists specific amounts in various food items.

What are the only three commonly available fruits native to North America?

40 High-Fiber Foods

Food group	Specific food	Serving size	Grams of dietary fiber
Breads	oat bran muffin	1 medium	2
	whole wheat bread	1 slice	2
	rye bread	1 slice	2
	raisin bread	1 slice	1
Cereals	Kellogg's All-Bran® (with Extra Fiber)	1/2 cup	14
	General Mills Fiber One®	1/2 cup	13
	Post Fruit and Fibre®	1/2 cup	5
	Kellogg's Raisin Bran®	3/4 cup	5
	General Mills Total®	1 cup	3
	Nabisco Shredded Wheat®	1 biscuit	3
	General Mills Wheaties®	1 cup	3
	Post Grape-Nuts®	1/4 cup	3
	Quaker Oatmeal®	1 packet	2–3
Fruits	dried apricots	1/4 cup	6
	dried dates	5	4
	dried prunes	3	4
	blackberries	1/2 cup	4
	orange	1	3
	apple (with skin)	1 (medium)	3
	strawberries	3/4 cup	3
	grapefruit	1/2	2.5
	banana	1 (medium)	2
	tangerine	1	2
Legumes (cooked)	kidney beans	1/2 cup	9
	baked beans	1/2 cup	7
	pinto beans	1/2 cup	5
	lentils	1/2 cup	2
Nuts	almonds	25	3
	walnuts	1/4 cup	2
	peanut butter	1 tablespoon	1
Pasta	whole-wheat	1 cup	5
Vegetables	baked potato	1 (with skin)	4
	broccoli	1/2 cup cooked	3
	corn	1/2 cup cooked	3
	Brussels sprouts	1/2 cup cooked	2
	carrot	1 (medium) cooked	3
	green beans	1/2 cup cooked	2
	eggplant	1/2 cup cooked	2
	avocado	1/2 (medium)	2
	popcorn	1 cup	2

Recommendations

1. Avoid processed foods; they lack fiber.
2. In setting up your daily eating plan, make sure you choose items that will add up to give you 25 to 40 grams of fiber in your daily diet.
3. Recognize that raw fruits and vegetables are generally better sources of fiber than are cooked vegetables.
4. Frequently include oat-bran muffins, oatmeal, or oat-bran cereal in your breakfast.

Recommended Resources

The American Red Cross' course Better Eating for Better Health (call your local chapter).

For people on the go, one packet of FibreSonic® or one Matola™ bar from Matol (800-237-7002) provide approximately 11 grams of dietary fiber.

Favorite Reading

Berkeley Wellness Letter, University of California, issued monthly, Box 420148, Palm Coast, FL 32142.

Answer:

The blueberry, cranberry, and Concord grape

12

AVOID MIGRAINE TRIGGERS

Migraine headaches are more common than is generally appreciated, affecting an estimated 23 million Americans. Many migraines are brought on by foods, additives, or pollutants, and for many individuals the following list has proven extremely useful. If you have recurrent, throbbing, or pulsating "vascular" headaches, perhaps with visual changes, perhaps with nausea and vomiting ("sick headaches"), perhaps worsened by bright light, generally relieved by sleep, and if you and your physician have ruled out other medical causes, use this list. See if you can identify specific triggers that you have ingested or experienced in the preceding 12 hours. Check the ingredient label on foods carefully for specific additives, for example, MSG (monosodium glutamate) to which some people are especially sensitive.

A related, but distinct category of vascular headaches is that of caffeine-withdrawal headaches. These differ from migraines in that they appear 24–48 hours after *stopping* caffeine, and are a withdrawal phenomenon.

I. Foods That May Trigger Migraines

Alcohol:	Sour cream	Pickled/marinated foods
Red/White wine	Nuts/peanut butter	Pizza
Champagne	Beans/pea pods	Excessive coffee or tea
Vodka	Processed meats	Monosodium glutamate
Rum	(with pork):	("Accent"®)
Liqueurs	Hot dogs	Onions/garlic (in excess)
Beer	Salami	Diet sodas/Nutrasweet®
Cheese:	Ham	Avocado
Cheddar	Bologna	Vitamins A, D, E, Niacin
Brie	Bacon	Artificial food coloring
Stilton	Sausage	Artificial food flavorings
Camembert	Chocolate	Preservatives
Blue	Bananas	(especially BHT, BHA)
Yogurt	Herring	

II. Other Factors
That May Trigger Migraines

Smoke (especially menthol cigarettes)
Long car trips (worse with smoker in car)
Fumes from paints, gasoline, paint thinner, car exhaust, cleaning
    fluid, varnish, Varathane®

	Missing a meal
Birth-control pills	Excessive noise
Sunlight	Too much sleep
High altitude	Smog
Fluorescent lights	Emotional stress
Hormone pills	Onset of menstruation
Perfume	Pregnancy

(This list is adapted from one provided by Allan Bernstein, M.D., neurologist, Kaiser Permanente Medical Center, Hayward, California; used with permission).

Recommendations

1. Use the above list to pinpoint whether specific foods or food additives are migraine triggers for you.
2. Wear tinted lenses to cut down on sunlight and fluorescent lights.
3. Avoid smoke, smog, fumes, and other irritants.
4. Exercise regularly (see Chapter 1).
5. Get the right amount of sleep for you (see Chapter 2).
6. Reduce the amount of stress in your life (see Chapter 33).
7. If you are on medication and are having migraines, ask your doctor to help you try other brands or generic forms of the medication. Frequently, the problem is not with the actual medicine, but with the supposedly inert and neutral materials used to make up the bulk of the tablet, capsule, or syrup.
8. Eat right, eat regularly, eat carefully.

Recommended Resource

The National Headache Foundation: 800-843-2256. Call for free brochures or physician referrals.

Favorite Reading

Migraine: Understanding a Common Disorder, by Oliver Sacks, M.D. Berkeley: University of California Press, 1985, 270 pgs.

Answer:

Cow's milk, eggs, soybeans, chocolate, peanuts,
shell fish, pork, tomatoes, corn, and wheat (gluten)

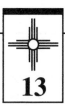

13

KNOW YOUR PERCENTAGE OF BODY FAT

Considerable national attention about twins and obesity was generated by an article in *The New England Journal of Medicine* in the early 1990s. In an effort to better understand whether heredity or environment is more important in determining body weight, researchers studied more than 650 pairs of twins. The proportion of their eventual adult body size that was controlled by their heredity (genes) was calculated to be 70%!

The 1991 book *The Great Divide* reported that "60 million females and 41 million males are on a diet on an average day!" Obviously, diets alone are seldom the answer. In fact, crash diets and wide fluctuations in body weight are *hazardous* to your health. Another medical report recently showed that the two factors that helped most with weight loss over long periods of time were *praise* and *exercise*. That is, people who are physically active and are praised for trying to lose weight lose more weight than do people who are inactive and whose efforts are not acknowledged.

Choosing a Realistic Weight Goal

Rather than refer to standardized weight charts, we would recommend that you utilize your percentage of body fat. We probably all know people whose weight is "normal" but who are out of shape and have too much fat. On the other hand, Covert Bailey's *Fit or Fat* describes zealous athletes who have overtrained to the point that they have too little body fat, and thus have reduced their stamina. Many adults who think they are "too fat" may in fact not be. Find a place to get your body fat measured and followed. The classic method of measuring body fat has been underwater immersion. Nearly as accurate, and much more convenient, are the computerized electrical resistance machines. They can be found at

Which state recently passed a requirement that
high-school wrestlers maintain at least 7% body fat?

33

some cardiac rehabilitation labs, metabolic clinics, and health fairs. Getting your body fat measured is well worth the $5 to $40 that it costs, and the information you get is more useful than what you see when you step on your bathroom scale.

Percentages of Body Fat

	Men	Women
Normal range for adults (20–45 yrs.)	6–20%	9–25%
Normal range for adults (over 45 yrs.)	6–24%	9–30%
Optimal fitness range	12–18%	16–25%
Obesity	Over 25%	Over 30%

Recommendations

1. Choose friends who give you direct praise and positive feedback for your healthy nutritional choices and the results. Let them know that you are working on weight control.
2. Begin, or continue, a regular exercise program (see Chapter 1).
3. Beware especially of saturated animal fats; limit these to 10% of total daily calories.
4. Try drinking 6 to 8 glasses of water per day.
5. Consume more fiber (see Chapter 11), which is filling but largely *indigestible*.
6. Have your body fat percent measured; you may be less "fat" than you think.
7. Learn to accept the genes and body build with which you were born.

Recommended Resource

For clinics interested in measuring body fat, Futrex has one of the best products (800-638-8739).

Favorite Readings

Overcoming Overeating, by Jane Hirschmann and Carol Munter. Reading, MA: Addison-Wesley, 1988, 259 pgs.

Great Shape: The First Fitness Guide for Large Women, by Pat Lyons and Debby Burgard. Palo Alto, CA: Bull Publishing, 1990, 242 pgs.

Answer:

Wisconsin

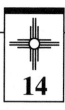

14

KNOW YOUR
FAMILY HEALTH HISTORY

Some people have a strong intuitive sense of how they will die. One man might say, "My dad died of a heart attack, my uncle died of a heart attack, and my grandfather died of a heart attack. I think I know what will do me in." Keeping his cholesterol low and staying physically active might be high priorities for him.

Why Know Your Family History?

Early in 1990 actor Gene Wilder gave a touching television interview about the recent death of his wife, Gilda Radner, formerly a star on *Saturday Night Live*. Ms. Radner died of ovarian cancer. She had been having vague symptoms and thought cancer might be the cause. When she sought medical advice, she was incorrectly reassured that there was no cancer. Ten months later, when the cancer was diagnosed, it had already spread to her liver, and she eventually died from it. More recently, Mr. Wilder disclosed that Gilda's grandmother, her aunt, and her cousin had all suffered from ovarian cancer, a fact of which she was unaware.

Sometimes you may hear someone say that his or her mother died of "kidney trouble." Such a term might have been used in explaining to the family what had happened. But it isn't precise enough to help the person define the family health history, or to anticipate his or her own likely medical problems. The mother could have died of chronic diabetes, bacterial infection of the kidneys, an immune disease, "shock kidney" because of a bullet wound, end-stage high-blood-pressure renal disease, cancer of the kidneys, or other possibilities. You need to know the precise cause of death in order to know what you need to be on guard against.

Your Family Health Record

Family member	Year of birth	Known medical conditions	Year of death	Cause of death
Paternal Grandfather				
Paternal Grandmother				
Maternal Grandfather				
Maternal Grandmother				
Father				
Mother				
Brother				
Brother				
Sister				
Sister				

Recommendations

1. Discuss with your living relatives what conditions and diseases "run in the family" for all immediate relatives (parents, brothers, sisters, children) and second-degree relatives (grandparents, uncles, aunts, nephews, nieces).
2. Where there are gaps in the medical information, track down hospital records and death certificates.
3. People who were adopted can petition for medical information.
4. Make an appointment with your personal physician specifically to go over your family health history with you, and make sure that this information is in your medical chart.
5. If a particular illness runs in your family, find out what specific tests and screening should be included in your future health care (for example, CA 125 blood test for ovarian cancer).
6. Use the Family Health Record on this page to help yourself gather your family's medical history. Go over this information with your physician at your next check-up.

Favorite Reading

The best book we have found for organizing your family's medical history is *MarLor's Family Health Record* (St. Paul, MN: MarLor Press, 1989), 96 pgs. To order, call 800-669-4908.

Answer:
One in two

15

FIND A PHYSICIAN WHO MODELS HEALTHY BEHAVIOR

Several years ago a mother took her child for an exam at a pediatric clinic, after having just had a physical herself. Upon seeing her child's physician, she announced, "I'm never going back to that person again. That person smokes!" It was strikingly clear what impact modeling healthy behavior can have on adults as well as children.

Health surveys of physicians during recent years have shown that physicians don't always practice what they preach. Finding a doctor who takes good care of himself or herself can be a valuable part of your strategy for taking good care of your own health. The next time you go in for your medical check-up, you might ask your health-care provider when was the last time that he or she had a physical.

"Find a physician you can pin down," advises one health-care consumer from El Paso, Texas. Know what questions are important to you when you go in for your office visit. Make sure you get answers that are clear enough for you to understand. Sometimes the most honest answer is, "I don't know."

Think out in advance the questions you have for your doctor, so that you can get the most out of your office visit. Write your questions down and prioritize them. Let your doctor know at the very beginning of your visit how many concerns you have, so that you can both deal with them as efficiently as possible.

Recommendation

Find a physician or nurse practitioner with whom you can relate well, whom you can trust, and whom you respect.

Favorite Reading

Harvard Health Letter (issued monthly), Subscription Dept., Box 420299, Palm Coast, FL 32142-9858.

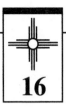

16

KNOW THE SEVEN WARNING SIGNS OF CANCER

Paradoxically, as health care improves and Americans in general live longer, your chances of developing and dying from cancer increase. In this area, as with the rest of your health, there is plenty you can do to increase the odds in your favor.

In 1991 there appeared a report that the gene thought to be responsible for cancer of the colon and rectum had been identified. This is potentially a very important discovery. Currently, more than 150,000 adults each year develop this disease, which ranks high among total cancer deaths. Previous reports have already linked specific genes with lung cancer and breast cancer. Check with your physician periodically on the practical developments in this emerging field of "cancer genes."

According to "Healthy People 2000," approximately 30% of cancer deaths are linked to smoking, and another 35% are associated with diet!

Current Top Seven Cancer Deaths by Site, from American Cancer Society's 1991 Estimates

	Men	Women
1.	Lung 34%	Lung 21%
2.	Prostate 12%	Breast 18%
3.	Colon/Rectum 11%	Colon/Rectum 13%
4.	Leukemia/Lymphomas 8%	Leukemia/Lymphomas 7%
5.	Bladder/Kidney 5%	Pancreas 5%
6.	Pancreas 4%	Ovary 5%
7.	Stomach 3%	Uterus (Womb) and Cervix .4%

The American Cancer Society's
Seven Warning Signs of Cancer

- Change in bowel or bladder habits.
- A sore that does not heal.
- Unusual bleeding or discharge.
- Thickening or lump in breast or elsewhere.
- Indigestion or difficulty in swallowing.
- Obvious change in wart or mole.
- Nagging cough or hoarseness.

Recommendations

1. Quit smoking.
2. Know your family medical history.
3. Take advantage of the appropriate screening tests: yearly Pap smears for women, mammograms, flexible sigmoidoscopic exams after age 50, etc. (However, routine chest X-rays for lung cancer are not generally recommended unless you are a smoker or have an occupational exposure history, such as to asbestos.)
4. Avoid passive smoke.
5. Eat more bran and fiber. Low-fat, high-fiber diets decrease the risk of colorectal and several other cancers.
6. Get a complete physical exam every 1–3 years from age 20 on, depending on your age and as recommended by your physician. For males this is helpful in detecting early prostate cancer.
7. Use sunscreen and *avoid getting sunburned.*
8. Have your house tested for radon gas if you live in a high-risk area. (Check with your local Health Department.)
9. Be aware of unnecessary exposures to electromagnetic fields. The Environmental Protection Agency's *EMF Report* suggests a possible link to leukemia, lymphoma, and brain cancer. This doesn't mean you have to throw away your electric blanket, but you might want to use it to warm up your bed, then turn it off (and unplug it) and add a comforter. (See *Nature,* June 7, 1990, or the *Harvard Health Letter,* March 1990.)
10. Avoid excessive exposure to those heavy metals known to cause cancer: radium, arsenic, lead, nickel, and chromium.
11. Consider cutting back red-meat consumption to once a week or less.
12. Precook foods to be barbecued in a microwave (80%), pour off the fats, then finish cooking on a grill.
13. Reduce saturated fat intake to 10% of your daily caloric total.
14. Know the seven warning signs of cancer.

Summary of American Cancer Society Recommendations for the Early Detection of Cancer in Asymptomatic People

Test or Procedure	Population		
	Sex	Age	Frequency
Sigmoidoscopy	M & F	50 and over	Every 3 to 5 years based on advice of physician
Stool Guaiac Slide Test	M & F	Over 50	Every year
Digital Rectal Examination	M & F	Over 40	Every year
Pap Test	F		All women who are or who have been sexually active, or have reached age 18, should have an annual Pap test and pelvic examination. After a woman has had three or more consecutive satisfactory normal annual examinations, the Pap test may be performed less frequently at the discretion of her physician.
Pelvic Exam	F	18–40 Over 40	Every 1–3 years with Pap test every year
Endometrial Tissue Sample	F	At menopause, women at high risk*	At menopause
Breast Self-examination	F	20–40	Every month
Breast Physical Examination	F	20–40 Over 40	Every 3 years Every year
Mammography & Cancer Check-up**	F	35–39 40–49 50 & over	Baseline Every 1–2 years Every year

* History of infertility, failure to ovulate, abnormal uterine bleeding, or estrogen therapy.

**To include examination for cancers of the thyroid, testicles, prostate, ovaries, lymph nodes, oral region, and skin.

Reproduced with permission of Dr. Gerald Dodd, Dr. Curtis Mettlin, J.B. Lippincott company, & American Cancer Society.

Recommended Resources

1. For prevention and treatment programs, call Cancer Information Service, 800-422-6237.
2. American Cancer Society, 800-ACS-2345.
3. To consult with registered dieticians regarding nutrition questions and a dietary guideline, call the American Institute for Cancer, 800-843-8114.
4. For information regarding hospice care, call or write The Hospice Education Institute, 5 Essex Sq., Box 713, Essex, CT 06426-0713, 800-544-2213.

Favorite Reading

American Cancer Society's pamphlet *What It Is* (especially pages 4 and 5 *Safeguards*), 90 Park Avenue, New York, NY 10016.

17

CARE FOR YOUR BREASTS

Women of any age, and even men, can develop breast cancer. But the group that has the most to gain from paying careful attention to their breasts is women between 30 and 80. The most reliable method of detecting breast cancer *at an early stage* is a mammogram, an X-ray of the breasts.

"The whole point of mammography is that you can find the breast cancer two years before you can feel it," says Cori Vancheri, director of the National Cancer Institute's early-detection education program. And the radiation exposure from a mammogram is less than that received going through an airport weapons detector, according to Dr. Daniel Kopans, director of breast imaging at Massachusetts General Hospital.

Statistics

- Breast cancer is the most frequent and second most deadly cancer among women in this country.
- An estimated 175,000 women will be diagnosed with breast cancer in the coming year.
- Approximately 44,000 women will die from this disease this year.
- According to an early 1990s Center for Health Statistics report, among U.S. women 40 and older, only 64% have *ever* had a mammogram, and only 15% have had one in the last year.

Recommendations

1. For adult women, learn how to perform a breast self-exam, and do one every month. For a plastic card to hang in your shower showing how to do a breast self-exam, call the Komen Alliance Clinical Breast Center, 800- I'M AWARE or 214-820-2430.

What is the risk of an American woman developing breast cancer in her lifetime?

2. For women 40 or over, get an annual breast exam by your health-care provider. Younger women should be checked at least every three years.
3. As recommended by the American Cancer Society, get an initial mammogram at age 40, then every 1 to 2 years from 40 to 50, and every year after 50. If you have a personal history of breast cancer or a positive family history of breast cancer, you may need earlier or more frequent mammograms.
4. Stop smoking. You will reduce your chances of getting breast cancer by 10 to 20%.
5. Eat a high-fiber diet.

Recommended Resources

American Cancer Society, 800-ACS-2345.

Y-ME-National Organization for breast cancer information and support, 708-799-8228.

Favorite Reading

Dr. Susan Love's Breast Book, by Susan Love, M.D., and Karen Lindsey. Reading, MA: Addison-Wesley, 1990, 455 pgs.

Answer:
1 in 9

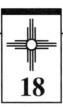

18

IMMUNIZE YOURSELF

Many of us think of shots as being just for kids. The fact is that there are approximately fifteen immunizations available today that are intended for adults. Several of these, such as those against yellow fever, typhoid, and cholera, are specifically intended for international travelers. Others, such as the rabies vaccine, are for those who may have special job-related risks. The other immunizations are available for adults regardless of occupation or travel plans; take advantage of those that apply to your age and risk groups.

Eradication of Smallpox

One of the greatest success stories in medicine has been the eradication in this century of smallpox throughout the world. The last case of non-laboratory smallpox occurred in Somalia in 1977. In the last ten years, there has not been a single natural case reported. The World Health Organization and thousands of health-care workers achieved this goal after a vigorous immunization campaign. Many Americans still have a scar on their shoulder from a smallpox vaccine received years ago.

Statistics and Recent Developments

- Fewer than half of Americans over 60 have up-to-date tetanus immunizations.
- Every year, almost 2 million children worldwide still die from measles; that's almost 3 deaths a minute! In the U.S., the number of measles cases reported in 1989 was a 400% increase over the year before, and 1990 saw another 50% increase.
- Several flu epidemics in this country in recent decades have each caused more than ten thousand deaths.
- There are 300,000 new cases of hepatitis B each year in the U.S.
- Only four cases of polio were reported in the Western Hemisphere in the first eight months of 1991!
- The year 2000 has been targeted by the World Health Organization for the worldwide eradication of polio. Rotary International has committed more than $200 million toward this effort.

Which common childhood disease still kills nearly 2,000,000 children worldwide each year?

Recommendations

1. Get a tetanus/diphtheria booster every ten years. If you get a dirty wound or laceration more than five years after your last booster, you'll need another tetanus shot.
2. Get a flu shot in the fall if you: are 65 or older; have heart, lung, or other chronic disease; are an insulin-dependent diabetic; are a health-care worker or resident of a chronic-care facility; are HIV positive or have AIDS; are under 18 years old and on long-term aspirin therapy.
3. Get the hepatitis B vaccine series if you are a health-care worker in contact with blood products.
4. If you are one of the 150,000 Americans suffering from hepatitis C, ask your physician about the recently approved interferon injections.
5. Get a measles booster if you are a teenager, college student, or health-care worker having direct patient contact, or if you were born after 1956.
6. If you are pregnant, get your blood tested to see if you have adequate immunity against rubella.
7. Have a skin test every 5 to 10 years to see if you have been exposed to tuberculosis.
8. If you are 65 or older (many internists say 55 or older) get a pneumococcal vaccine to prevent pneumonia.
9. Consider a polio booster if you are traveling to a third-world country.
10. Consult with your health-care provider if you're planning a trip out of the country.

Recommended Resource

Centers for Disease Control Disease Information Hotline, Atlanta, GA, 404-332-4559.

Favorite Reading

The Medical Detectives, by Berton Roueche. New York: Truman Talley Books/Plume, 1991, 421 pgs.

Answer:
Measles

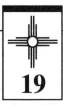

19

TAKE AN ASPIRIN EVERY OTHER DAY

Heart attacks and heart disease are the number-one cause of death in this country with more than half a million adults dying from heart disease each year. For years, physicians and scientists have investigated ways of using the blood-thinning properties of aspirin to reduce this risk. A proven strategy has been developed.

Aspirin Research in Men

In 1981, Harvard Medical School began a national study in which more than 22,000 male physicians, ages 40–84, were followed for heart attacks. Women were not included at that time, largely because their rates of heart disease prior to menopause were much lower, so that any benefits of the experiment would have taken longer to prove. Half the men participating took one adult aspirin every other day; the other half took a placebo or sugar pill. An analysis was done each year. After four-and-a-half years, the study was halted. Those in the aspirin group had suffered 139 heart attacks, with 10 heart-attack deaths; the placebo group had 239 heart attacks and 26 heart-attack deaths.

Benefits for Women

The risk of heart attacks for women has increased in recent years as smoking rates among women have increased, and as women pursue more stressful careers and lifestyles. Evidence is now emerging that women also may benefit from preventive doses of aspirin. Results of a large study of 87,000 nurses demonstrated a 30% lowering of heart-attack risk for those on aspirin according to a report given at an American Heart Association conference in the early 1990s.

What percent of Europeans who have had one heart attack are reported to be on low-dose aspirin therapy?

Dangers of Aspirin Use

The side effects of regular aspirin use are significant. Because aspirin reduces blood clotting, bleeding is more likely, and bleeding time is lengthened. There are increased chances of nosebleeds, gastrointestinal bleeding, ulcer disease, increased wheezing in some asthmatics, hemorrhage in the eyes, and some strokes. If there is a significant history of hemorrhagic strokes in your family medical history, taking aspirin every other day may not be for you. *Discuss the risks and benefits with your physician.* Because of the blood-clotting problems, it's preferable not to take aspirin for the ten days prior to any scheduled surgery.

Recommendation

If you are over 50 and don't have medical reasons for not taking aspirin, you can lessen your risk of a heart attack by taking one adult aspirin every other day. Taking a buffered or coated form of aspirin will reduce the risk of gastrointestinal side effects. And adults who have had *one* heart attack can definitely lower their odds of a *second* heart attack with low-dose aspirin every other day.

Favorite Reading

The report of the U.S. Preventive Services Task Force, published as *The Guide to Clinical Preventive Services*: *An Assessment of the Effectiveness of 169 Interventions*. Baltimore, MD: Williams and Wilkins, 1989, 419 pgs.

Addendum: Another unexpected benefit of frequent aspirin use has been a decrease by 40% in deaths from cancer of the colon. Since this research was supervised by the American Cancer Society, and involved more than 662,000 subjects, it is hard to dismiss the findings as mere chance. Doctors do not yet have a full explanation for this latest benefit from regular aspirin usage.

Answer:
90%

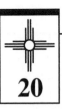

20

PERFECT THE HEIMLICH MANEUVER

Several years ago, a famous New Orleans physician began choking on food while attending a banquet with dozens of other doctors. He excused himself from his table and went alone to the men's room, rather than seeking help or "causing a scene." He died from obstruction of his airway.

Many of us may have been present when someone was choking on food, usually on a piece of meat, which the American Heart Association tells us accounts for about 3,000 deaths each year. One waitress in Florida is reported to have saved four people in one month from choking emergencies. It would help us all to know the universal signal that means "I am choking on food," and to learn the Heimlich maneuver, so that we can propel an object out of somebody else's upper airway in an emergency.

Performing the Heimlich maneuver

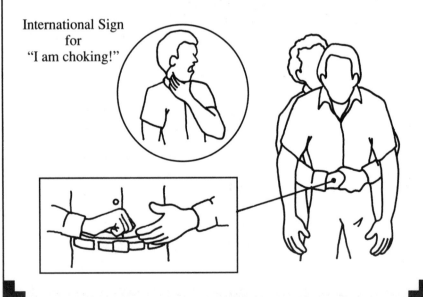

International Sign for "I am choking!"

After about how many minutes without oxygen do the cells of the brain begin to die?

Stand behind the choking person, clasp your hands with the knuckle of your thumbs underneath his or her rib cage as shown above, and thrust toward yourself quickly. If the person is lying on the ground, kneel down, and use your straightened arms to create a thrust under the person's ribs.

The Heimlich maneuver can cause rib and internal injury. Do not practice on another person. Use this technique only if a person is really choking.

Recommendations

1. Know both the signal that means "I am choking on food," and the Heimlich maneuver. Make sure that other members of your household also know these skills.
2. Realize that you may well panic if someone you love is choking! Ask the American Red Cross for their posters "When an Adult Is Choking" and "When a Child Is Choking." Hang these in your kitchen or somewhere obvious to remind yourself, babysitters, or others in your home how to respond to a choking emergency.
3. Practice the technique with your family and have them practice it with you, using only *gentle* force so you don't break someone's ribs.
4. If you are alone and choking, you can perform the maneuver on yourself by clasping your hands and thrusting upward under your rib cage. Alternatively, you may dislodge the obstruction by throwing yourself over the back of a sofa or armchair to create a thrust just below your rib cage.
5. Sign up for a CPR (cardiopulmonary resuscitation) course through your local American Heart Association or American Red Cross, and encourage your family to join you.

Recommended Resource

Wallet-sized cards demonstrating the Heimlich maneuver are available from Edumed, Inc., Box 52, Cincinnati, OH 45201, or from your local American Red Cross chapter.

Favorite Reading

Mayo Clinic Health Letter, c/o Mayo Clinic, 200 1st St., S.W., Rochester, MN 55905.

Answer:
Four minutes

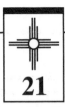

21

BE ACCIDENT ALERT

Accidents are among the top ten leading causes of death for those over 60 in this country, and more than half these accidents involve falls. It isn't always the fall itself that does you in; it's often the prolonged convalescence resulting from the fall. The following list of recommendations applies to most adults and especially to older Americans. Use them to safeguard both your home and your health.

Recommendations

1. Get enough calcium in your daily diet to preserve your bone strength (see Chapter 8).
2. Have your vision checked every one to two years.
3. Use a shower mat or tub strips that are designed to prevent slipping.
4. Use night lights in the hallway, bathroom, and bedroom to prevent falls at night.
5. Throw away throw rugs.
6. Use handrails wherever they would be helpful. Put them in your stairways, in your showers, and next to your bathtub.
7. Use rubber tips for the bottom of any canes or walking sticks; tips that won't slip on ice are especially useful.
8. Install a shelf for packages near the doorway to your home.
9. Add abrasive strips to the front edge of your outside steps.
10. Paint your top and bottom steps white, so that they will be more easily visible. Most falls on stairs involve the top or the next-to-the-bottom step.
11. Lower the temperature of your water heater (110–120°) to reduce the chance of burns when showering.
12. Install a smoke alarm on each floor of your home.
13. *Never* smoke in bed.
14. Make sure your fire extinguishers are still functional.
15. Make sure your shoes fit properly.
16. Use a step stool with *sturdy* handrails to reach overhead items.
17. Walk and exercise regularly. A report in the *Journal of the American Medical Association* showed that 90% of ninety year olds increased their muscle strength from 10 to 50% within eight weeks through a supervised exercise program!

18. Regularly discuss any medication with your doctor to be sure it is still appropriate for your weight, liver, and kidney function. In addition, discuss your various medications to make sure they don't cross-react with one another.
19. Consider wearing a MedAlert® bracelet listing major diseases (such as diabetes), any drug allergies, and essential medications. Call the Medic Alert Foundation (800-432-5378).
20. Look into the communication systems for older citizens concerned about getting help if they should have a bad fall or loss of consciousness. Two of the best available are Lifeline Systems (800-543-5346) and MedicAlert® Response Service (800-423-6333).
21. Fill out a Durable Power of Attorney for Health Care (see Chapter 22).
22. Wear a helmet when riding a bicycle: it will protect you and will be good modeling for your children and grandchildren.
23. Use timers on lights in your home, so that you don't have to walk into a dark house.
24. Buy a portable telephone to avoid rushing to a distant receiver.
25. Have your adult children buy and read Joan Levin's sensitive *How to Care for Your Parents* (Washington, DC: Storm King Press, 1987).

Recommended Videos

Positive Moves by Angela Lansbury, an exercise tape for adults over 50.

55 Alive, c/o American Association of Retired Persons, 1909 K St. N.W., Washington, DC 20049 (co-sponsored by General Motors Corp.) on defensive driving skills.

Favorite Reading

80 Dos and 50 Don'ts for Your Safety: A Practical Guide for Eldercare, free from The Veterans Administration Geriatric Research, Education, and Clinical Center, 16111 Plummer St., Sepulveda, CA 91343, 16 pgs.

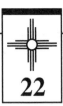

22

HAVE A DURABLE POWER OF ATTORNEY FOR HEALTH CARE

Most of us think of life-support systems, such as breathing machines and feeding tubes, as being primarily for the elderly. This is usually true, but not always. In fact *younger adults*, if they wish to not be artificially kept alive, may have the most to lose by not having their wishes documented in writing regarding life-support systems and catastrophic care.

Why Is a Durable Power of Attorney for Health Care Important?

References to Durable Power of Attorney for Health Care (DPAHC) documents are appearing more frequently in the media, due in part to the June 1990 Supreme Court decision regarding Nancy Cruzan. This unfortunate Missouri woman was left comatose after a 1983 car crash. At the time she was 25 years old. Until December 1990, she had been in a coma for nearly eight years, and was kept alive only because of a feeding tube surgically implanted in her stomach. After several years her parents made the difficult decision to ask that the support be removed, and that their daughter be allowed to die. Ms. Cruzan had expressed her wish, prior to the accident, not to be kept alive if she wasn't "half-way independent." But because she had not put her wishes in writing, several courts, including the state court and the U.S. Supreme Court, ruled that she should continue to be artificially fed, despite her parents' request. She subsequently died in late 1990.

What is the average monthly cost of being cared for in a permanent comatose state?

Background

- Less than 10% of American adults have a Durable Power of Attorney for Health Care in effect. These documents allow you to decide, while you are of sound mind, whom you might wish to appoint as your "proxy" to assure that physicians will carry out your express wishes, should you be unable to speak for yourself. Such wishes can include *refusing* various treatments.
- Currently, 41 states and the District of Columbia have "living will laws" allowing patients to decline prolonged life-support, and 22 states and the District of Columbia recognize Durable Power of Attorney for Health Care laws. Some have both. Some have neither.
- Living wills have four features that differ from DPAHC:
    1. Most do not specifically designate a proxy.
    2. Requests pertain only to forgoing life support.
    3. Most apply only if you are terminally ill.
    4. Physicians who follow these documents may not be legally protected in so doing.
- As of December 1991, the federal Patient Self-Determination Act mandates that hospitals be sure that all patients are aware of their right to complete an "advance directive."
- Approximately *ten thousand* people in this country are in prolonged comas, sometimes referred to as "a persistent vegetative state," which can continue for 30 years or more.

Recommendations

1. If you do not want a prolonged, vegetative state imposed on you in the event of a coma-producing illness or accident, act now to make your wishes known *in writing*! Documents known as "advance directives" will help accomplish this. The most comprehensive is known as the "Durable Power of Attorney for Health Care."
2. Discuss your decisions and any questions you might have with your physician.
3. Make sure you give a copy of your "advance directive" to your proxy and your physician, and that you provide one for your medical chart.

4. Discuss your views about life support with family members, especially what quality of life would not be bearable.
5. While facing this difficult topic, also give some thought to being an organ donor at the time of your death. There are thousands of patients in this country waiting for an available organ donation.
6. Check with your state medical society or state bar association to make sure which forms are recognized in your state, and where to obtain them.

Recommended Resources

Choice in Dying, 250 W. 57th St., New York, NY 10107, 212-246-6962.

A sample copy of a Durable Power of Attorney for Health Care is available for $4.00 and appeared in the June 1990 issue of *The Harvard Medical School Health Letter*, Dept. B.I., P.O. Box 380, Boston, MA 02117.

Favorite Reading

The Power of Attorney Book, by Denis Clifford. Berkeley, CA: Nolo Press, 1991, 200 pgs.

Your Legal Rights in Later Life, by John Regan, J.S.D. Glenview, IL: Scott, Foresman, 1989, 321 pgs.

Answer:
$5,000–$6,000/month

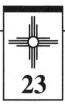

23

BE FIRST-AID PREPARED

Natural disasters can happen anywhere. These include hurricanes, typhoons, earthquakes, fires, and floods. If you're caught in one of these disasters, you'll need to be first-aid prepared. And illnesses and injuries can occur every day for both you and your family. Your medicine cabinet or supply cupboard should be stocked with the following supplies for any emergency. In addition, you'll need a several-day supply of water and all essential medications that members of your family use regularly.

- [ ] Ace bandages
- [ ] Adhesive tape
- [ ] Analgesics (aspirin or acetaminophen, e.g., Tylenol®)
- [ ] Antacids (e.g., Maalox®)
- [ ] Antibiotic ointment (e.g., Neosporin®)
- [ ] Antidiarrheal medicine (e.g., Imodium®, Pepto Bismol®)
- [ ] Antihistamines (for allergic reactions/itching; e.g., Benadryl®)
- [ ] Anti-itch lotion or spray (e.g., Calamine®)
- [ ] Bandaids
- [ ] Decongestants (e.g., Sudafed®)
- [ ] Epsom salts
- [ ] Foot powder or spray for athlete's foot
- [ ] Gauze dressing and bandages
- [ ] Hydrogen peroxide (3% solution)
- [ ] Petroleum jelly
- [ ] Rubbing alcohol
- [ ] Scissors
- [ ] Syrup of Ipecac (for poisonings)
- [ ] Thermometer
- [ ] Tweezers

In addition to the medical supplies listed on the previous page, you should have supplies and provisions set aside in case of a natural disaster. Each member of the household will need a *minimum* of eight ounces of water per day to last them for two to three days. In addition, you will need small amounts of non-thirst inducing food supplies. The following list is adapted from that provided by the American Red Cross.

- [ ] First Aid kit
- [ ] Blankets or sleeping bags
- [ ] Can opener
- [ ] Candles and matches, or light sticks
- [ ] Fire extinguisher
- [ ] Flashlight with fresh batteries
- [ ] Food supplies (1200+ calories per person per day)
- [ ] Gloves for clearing debris
- [ ] Medications (essential prescriptions)
- [ ] Pocket knife
- [ ] Prescription glasses
- [ ] Red Cross survival guide (see favorite reading)
- [ ] Spare shoes and clothing
- [ ] Transistor radio with batteries
- [ ] Watch or clock
- [ ] Water (distilled/bottled; 1–2 gallons for each household member)

Recommended Resource

Disaster Preparedness Products, by I.O.R., Inc., Kensington, CA; 510-528-3060.

Favorite Reading

American Red Cross "Family Disaster Plan and Survival Guide," 4 pgs., available from your local American Red Cross chapter.

Answer:

Cold water or ice

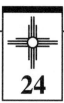

24

USE YOUR SEAT BELT

If you already use your seat belt every time you drive, keep it up. If you don't, start. This is the easiest change for better health that anyone in this country can make. Since motor-vehicle accidents are the fifth leading cause of death for adults of all ages, buckling up is statistically one of the most important things you can do for your health.

Why Seat Belts Are Important

- Motor-vehicle accidents kill more Americans ages 1 through 34 than any other cause of death.
- In California in 1988, 82% of those who died in motor-vehicle accidents were not wearing seat belts.
- Motor-vehicle accidents are the cause of 36% of all deaths at work!
- Wearing a seat belt is required by law in 36 states; in 8 states, you can be pulled over simply for not wearing one.
- Drivers protected by air bags are 4 to 7 times less likely to be seriously injured than are their front-seat passengers without one.
- For those who don't care to wear a seat belt, remember this: Bracing yourself with your arms in a 30-mph frontal crash is equivalent to catching a 300-pound bag of cement dropped from a second-storey window.

Surveys conducted at a Kaiser Permanente hospital in the San Francisco Bay Area over the last seven years reveal encouraging trends, as shown in the following table. The observations were made at various entrances to the hospital's parking areas. More than one thousand people were surveyed for each year reported.

Percentage of Drivers and Passengers Wearing Seat Belts

	1984	1985	1989	1990
Infants 0–4 years	63%	79%	81%	100%
Children 4–16 years	34	54	77	74
Adult visitors/patients	24	34	62	67
Staff	57	57	74	86
Physicians	84	80	92	90
Emergency depart. staff	not available			100
Totals	35%	43%	67%	75%

Adapted from Kaiser Pemanente Health Education surveys.

Why Should You Wear a Seat Belt?

Adapted from *Fairy Tales*, U.S. Department of Transportation, National Highway Traffic Safety Administration, Washington, DC 20590, February 1977.

1. "I don't need a safety belt when I'm traveling at low speeds or going on a short trip."

   All driving can be dangerous. More than 80% of all accidents occur at speeds less than 40 mph. Fatalities involving non-belted occupants of cars have been recorded at 12 mph, about the speed you'd be driving in a parking lot. Three out of four accidents causing death occur within 25 miles of home. Belt up before driving to your shopping center, just as you would for a long trip.

2. "I'm uncomfortable and too confined when I wear a safety belt."

   Belts are designed to allow you to reach necessary driving controls, and the newer shoulder-belt retractors give you even more freedom. When reaching for things that will take you away from the steering wheel, it's safer to pull off the road or ask your passenger to help. You'll probably find that any initial discomfort caused by safety belts soon goes away. Eventually, you may even feel more comfortable wearing safety belts.

3. "I might be saved if I'm thrown clear of the car in an accident."

Your chances of being killed are almost 25 times greater if you're thrown from the car. The forces in a collision can be great enough to fling you as much as 150 feet, or about 15 car lengths. Safety belts can keep you from:
- plunging through the windshield
- being thrown out the door and hurtled through the air
- scraping along the ground
- being crushed by your own car.

In almost any collision, you're better off being held inside the car by safety belts.

4. "If I wear a safety belt, I might be trapped in a burning or submerged car!"

Less than one-half of 1% of all injury-producing collisions involve fire or submersion. But if fire or submersion does occur, wearing a safety belt can save your life. If you're involved in a crash without your safety belt, you might be stunned or knocked unconscious by striking the interior of the car. Then your chances of getting out of a burning or submerged car would be far less. You're better off wearing a safety belt at all times in a car. With safety belts, you're more likely to be unhurt, alert, and capable of escaping quickly.

5. "It takes too much time and trouble to fasten my safety belt."

In reality, fastening your safety belt may take some time and trouble—but not too much. It all depends on:
- how complex your belt is
- how well you know how to use your belt
- how difficult it is to find the belt ends.

That much time and trouble you can live with, if you want to live.

6. "When I have my lap belt fastened, I don't need to fasten my shoulder belt."

A lap belt will protect you from serious injury, but a shoulder belt provides important additional protection. During a crash, a shoulder belt keeps your head and chest from striking the steering wheel, dashboard, and windshield. *A lap and shoulder belt offers you the best possible protection in the event of a crash.* A woman wearing only a shoulder belt was recently decapitated when she was entangled in the belt across her neck. This terrible event might have been prevented had she had on a lap belt, which would have held her in her seat.

Recommendation

Use your lap belt *and* shoulder belt every time you ride in a motor vehicle.

Favorite Reading

The Johns Hopkins Medical Letter *Health After 50*, Subscription Dept., Box 420179, Palm Coast, FL 32142

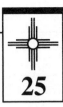

25

PROTECT YOUR SKIN FROM THE SUN

Did you ever wonder why senior golfers like Arnold Palmer and Chi Chi Rodriguez always wear hats on golf courses, whereas younger stars like Hale Irwin, Pattie Sheehan, Paul Azinger, and Robin Waterhouse only occasionally do? Perhaps golfers (and others) of a certain age realize the threat that continuous outdoor exposure poses to their skin.

The Threat from Ultraviolet Radiation

Many magazines and newspapers have had recent articles about the ozone layer, sunscreens, and skin cancer. As our ozone layer is diminished, more of the Sun's ultraviolet radiation reaches the Earth's surface, and with greater ultraviolet radiation comes a greater risk of skin cancer. As Dr. Perry Robbins, president of the Skin Cancer Foundation, says, "What cigarettes are to lung cancer, the sun is to skin cancer."

Currently 600,000 new cases of skin cancer are detected in the U.S. each year. More significantly, 8,000 people die each year from skin cancer, three-fourths of them from a type of skin cancer known as *malignant melanoma*. The other main types of skin cancer (squamous-cell carcinoma and basal-cell carcinoma) are more common, but less invasive and more easily treated. It is the recent *doubling* in cases of malignant melanoma that has attracted the most alarm and media attention.

Who Is Most at Risk for Melanoma?

- Women (one-and-a-half times more often than men)
- Adults over 40
- Outdoor workers
- Those with fair skin

What is the likelihood of an American adult developing skin cancer? 61

- Those with blond, red, or light brown hair, and those with blue, green, or grey eyes
- Those with a family history of malignant melanoma
- Adults with a history of severe or blistering sunburns
- Those with a large number of moles
- Young professionals who spend most of their time in offices and intermittently vacation or spend time in the sun
- Workers exposed to cancer-causing chemicals
- Those exposed to the Sun at high altitudes.

Know the ABCDs of Malignant Melanoma

A - Asymmetry: one half unequal to other half
B - Border irregularity: jagged, notched edges
C - Color: mottled variations in color
D - Diameter: greater than a pencil eraser.

Adapted from guidelines of the American Academy of Dermatology

Danger Signs in Moles

1. New moles
2. Enlarging moles
3. Change in color (especially red or black areas)
4. Itching or pain
5. Scaling of a mole
6. Bleeding or oozing from a mole
7. A new raised area within a mole.

The Good News about Skin Cancer

1. It's visible (unlike most other cancers)
2. It's curable (85 to 95% of the time)
3. It's preventable (with sunscreens).

And sunscreens not only lower your risk of skin cancer, they also decrease wrinkling and premature aging of your skin.

Recommendations

1. Avoid sunburn.
2. Plan your outdoor activities to avoid the peak sunlight hours from 10:00 a.m. to 3:00 p.m.
3. Use sunscreen with SPF (sun protection factor) of at least 15 (oil-free for teenagers and those with acne, oil-based for other adults).
4. Help your children avoid sunburn (50 to 80% of most people's lifetime Sun exposure occurs by age 20).
5. Tell your doctor about any skin lesion ("mole") that gets larger, bleeds, changes color, or becomes painful.
6. Use "broad-spectrum sunscreens," which protect against both type A and type B ultraviolet rays.
7. Wear waterproof sunscreen every day in sunny weather, as recommended by the National Institute of Health.
8. Avoid sunlamps and tanning booths.
9. Use sunscreening chapsticks to reduce the likelihood of lip cancer.
10. Consult your physician about medications that increase your sensitivity to ultraviolet light (the antibiotic tetracycline, oral birth-control pills, some blood-pressure medications).
11. To reduce wrinkling, consider Retin A (prescription required). However, it substantially increases sensitivity to ultraviolet light, so you'll need to use extra sunscreen protection.
12. To reduce dryness, use a moisturizing soap (e.g., Dove®) and lotion with sunscreen protection (e.g., Johnson and Johnson's Purpose®).
13. Wear polarized sunglasses to protect your eyes and eyelids.
14. If you have the risk factors listed above, especially a family history of malignant melanoma, have a complete skin exam by your doctor as often as recommended.
15. Know your skin (and its moles), and thoroughly examine it yourself every 1 to 6 months.

Recommended Resource

American Academy of Dermatology, *Melanoma Skin Cancer* brochure, 1567 Maple Ave., Evanston, IL 60201.

Favorite Reading

Sun Sense, by Perry Robbins, M.D. Skin Cancer Foundation, 245 Fifth Ave., Suite 2402, New York, NY 10016, 1990, 248 pgs.

Answer:
One in six (1 in 3 if you have fair skin and freckles)

26

BE AIDS AWARE

Just as bubonic plague and smallpox were dreaded diseases in past centuries, and as tuberculosis and polio were feared earlier in this century, so is AIDS feared today. AIDS (acquired immune deficiency syndrome) is usually fatal, treatments are only partially effective, and no vaccine is immediately in sight. A major difference, however, is that we understand how AIDS is spread, and, with proper precautions AIDS transmission can be prevented.

How to Avoid AIDS

We must know both how AIDS is and how it is *not* spread, so that we can avoid high-risk behaviors. Why do we need to know how AIDS is *not* spread? First, to reduce some of the hysteria centered around this disease. Second, to prevent unfair stigmatizing of AIDS patients when they are not a health risk to uninfected persons. AIDS is *not* spread by kissing, casual contact, mosquitoes, toilet seats, having a blood test, or donating blood. Nor is it likely, with the American Blood Bank screening tests currently in place, to be acquired by receiving a blood transfusion in the United States. Nor is it likely to be acquired from medical personnel who properly use "universal precautions" and proper sterilization techniques.

AIDS is spread by:
- Sharing drug needles or syringes
- Unprotected sexual intercourse with an infected partner
- Having received HIV-positive blood
- Being born to or breast-fed by an HIV-positive mother
- Accidental contact to broken skin or mucous membranes with infected blood or body fluids.
- Unsterilized ear-piercing or tattoo needles.

Being HIV Positive

Testing positive for HIV (human immune deficiency virus) is not the same as having AIDS. Being HIV positive means that you have been exposed to the AIDS virus, and have developed antibodies against it. Blood tests are available to make this diagnosis. After being exposed, it may be ten years or more before a person becomes sick with the disease of AIDS.

Some Facts about AIDS

- Right now, 1.5 million Americans are HIV positive, and 200,000 have AIDS.
- In 1989, more than 35,000 new cases of AIDS were officially reported.
- More than 1,300 American children have died from AIDS.
- 1 in 500 college students are currently infected with the AIDS virus, which translates into one member of the audience of a moderately full movie theater.
- There are currently 8 to 10 *million* men, women, and children with the AIDS virus worldwide.
- The World Health Organization projects that by the year 2000, there will be 30 million adults and an additional 10 million children with the AIDS virus.
- AIDS has often been considered a gay men's disease. But by the year 2000, 80% of new cases will be the result of heterosexual intercourse, or intravenous drug use.

Treatment and Prevention

For people infected with the AIDS virus, there are promising drugs available effective in slowing the progression of the disease, such as AZT, ddI, and ddC.

There are also other drugs such as pentamidine for treating the infections and complications associated with AIDS.

The Sixth International Conference on AIDS reported that a vaccine against AIDS is unlikely to be available before the year 2000.

At this time, education is the only "vaccine" we have against AIDS.

Recommendations

1. If you think there is any chance that you might have AIDS or be HIV positive, get tested! Clinics are available for free, anonymous testing, and counseling as well. Call your local hospital to locate available testing and resources near you.
2. Don't share needles and syringes.
3. Realize that unprotected sex is risky. A recent poll of college students showed that only 16% of female students and only 25% of male students used condoms during intercourse. Latex condoms largely reduce, but do not totally eliminate, the risk of acquiring AIDS.
4. Learn as much as you can about this tragic disease. Toll-free information number: National AIDS hotline, 800-342- AIDS; in Spanish, 800-344-7432; for hearing-impaired, 800-243-7889.

Favorite Reading

Risky Times, by Jeanne Blake. New York: Workman Publishing, 1990, 157 pgs.

Answer:
6 billion

27

KEEP YOUR SEX LIFE HEALTHY

Sexual involvements are rarely as straightforward as they first appear to be. This is especially true where health issues are concerned.

Some Facts about Sexually Transmitted Diseases (STDs)

There are more than 25 sexually transmitted diseases to which Americans are vulnerable. Younger women, in particular, have the most at stake when the risks of pregnancy and infertility are added to that of infection.

- There are 270,000 initial cases of genital herpes and 20 *million relapses* every year in this country.
- Syphilis cases were up 60% for the first half of 1990 over the year before, which had the highest incidence since 1949.
- Hepatitis B, which can be sexually transmitted, has infected between 500,000 and 1,000,000 Americans so far.
- There are 2 million new cases of gonorrhea every year.
- Every year there are 3 to 4 million new cases of chlamydia.
- The risk of ectopic pregnancy (where the fertilized egg attaches itself to the fallopian tube rather than inside the uterus) is doubled by chlamydia. Ectopic pregnancies, which are life-threatening for the mother, currently number 88,000 per year, which is a 20 to 25% increase *per year* since 1970!
- Pelvic inflammatory disease is a leading cause of infertility in hundreds of thousands of U.S. women.
- There are between 500,000 and *one million* pregnancies in unmarried teenagers each year. Between 80 and 90% of these are unintended.
- Approximately 400,000 of these pregnancies end in abortions.
- All of the above risks coexist with the increasing threat of AIDS (see Chapter 26).

What Is Safe Sex?

- Maintaining a mutually faithful monogamous sexual relationship with a non-infected partner
- Using latex condoms
- Abstaining from sexual intercourse.

Although latex condoms are estimated to be more than 90% effective in preventing transmission of the AIDs virus, they are not 100% effective.

Recommendations

1. Practice safe sex.
2. If you have been engaging in risky sexual behavior, get a thorough physical to find out if you are a carrier of any STD.

Recommended Resource

For local resources and further information, call the STD National Hotline, 800-227-8922.

Favorite Reading

Erotic Wars by Lillian Rubin. New York: Harper, 1991, 203 pgs.

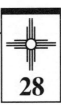

28

CONTROL YOUR BLOOD PRESSURE

High blood pressure has no symptoms. That is to say, you can be walking around with a very high blood pressure, for example 190/110, feel perfectly well, and die of a stroke the next day.

Why Is High Blood Pressure Dangerous?

High blood pressure is a contributing factor in three-fourths of heart attacks and strokes. Having higher than normal blood pressure puts a strain on your heart by increasing the pressure your heart must work against with each and every beat. Your chances of having a heart attack increase because of the extra strain. High blood pressure also means more pressure in the blood vessels in your brain. If one of them ruptures because of the pressure, you've had a stroke. Lowering your blood pressure to normal levels decreases the risk of these two permanently damaging, often fatal, conditions.

Particularly at high risk are people with a family history of high blood pressure, and those with already existing complications such as heart disease, stroke, or kidney impairment. Dr. Charles Johnson, president of the National Medical Association, reminds us that 50% of those with high blood pressure are unaware that they have hypertension. He also warns that high blood pressure is the single most devastating illness affecting African-Americans.

Degrees of Blood Pressure

	systolic/diastolic
Normal	120/80
Mildly high	140/90 or greater
Moderately high	160/105 or greater
Severely high	180/115 or greater

Recommendations

1. The good news is that you can do something about high blood pressure. Have your blood pressure checked by your health-care provider at least every 3 years. If it is too high, use the following ideas, and then have your blood pressure checked again in 1 to 6 months.
2. Get in shape (see Chapter 1).
3. Take more control over your day-to-day worklife (see Chapter 40).
4. Stop smoking (see Chapter 31).
5. Take a stress-reduction class.
6. Practice a meditation or relaxation technique daily (see Chapter 6).
7. Take blood-pressure medication as recommended by your doctor.
8. Use less sodium and salt (less than 2500 mgs. of sodium per day).
9. Moderate your alcohol intake (see Chapter 30).
10. Drink fewer than four cups of caffeinated coffee a day.
11. If you are pregnant, have your blood pressure checked each month at your prenatal checkups.

Favorite Reading

The Harvard Heart Letter, issued monthly, Box 420234, Palm Coast, FL 32142-0234.

Dr. Dean Ornish's Program for Reversing Heart Disease. New York: Random House, 1990, 631 pgs.

Answer:
75%

29

LOWER YOUR RISK OF A STROKE

Those of us who are old enough will probably remember Ruby Keeler, star of stage and screen, dancing her way through *No, No, Nanette,* and *42nd Street.* Recently, she has starred on television as the National Stroke Association's spokesperson, advising us to know the warning signs of a stroke. Ms. Keeler had a stroke in 1979, and today she speaks out so that others can avoid the devastating consequences of a stroke. The risk of a stroke can be reduced.

What Is a Stroke?

A stroke is the death of an area of nerve cells in the brain. These cells die because of a sudden loss of their blood supply. Strokes, which are also known as cerebral vascular accidents (CVAs), are the third most common cause of death in America, and the *leading* cause of adult disability. Know the warning signs of a stroke. By taking action, you may be able to avert a stroke, or at least reduce its severity.

Warning Signs of a Stroke

1. Sudden blurred or decreased vision in one or both eyes.
2. Numbness, weakness, or paralysis of the face, or in either an arm or a leg, on one or both sides of the body.
3. Difficulty in speaking or understanding.
4. Dizziness, loss of balance, or an unexplained fall.
5. Difficulty in swallowing.
6. Headache that is severe and comes on abruptly, or unexplained changes in a pattern of headaches.

These symptoms are usually temporary, and last from a few seconds up to 24 hours. After 24 hours you may think you have recovered. However, these episodes may be a mini-stroke caused by a temporary interruption in the blood supply to your brain. Do not ignore these signs. There may be a hidden problem in your circulatory system, and it could get worse. These temporary interruptions, known as TIAs (transient ischemic attacks), are serious warning signs of stroke. About half of stroke survivors have a history of these TIAs. See your doctor as to the necessity of further testing.

Risk Factors for a Stroke

A few risk factors for stroke are irreversible, but most of them can be eliminated or reduced by specific actions you can take, according to the National Stroke Association. The following risk factors are treatable medical disorders and life-style habits that can be changed:
- High blood pressure (the most important known risk factor)
- Smoking
- Cocaine, amphetamines, and heroin
- High cholesterol level
- Carotid artery narrowing (detectable by a physical exam)
- Heart disease, such as infected valves or atrial fibrillation, both of which are treatable
- Excessive alcohol consumption
- Obesity
- Oral contraceptives (especially for women over age 40)
- Poorly controlled diabetes
- Past TIAs.

Recommendations

1. Reduce your blood pressure if it is elevated (see Chapter 28).
2. Quit smoking (see Chapter 31).
3. Avoid dangerous drugs and excessive use of alcohol (see Chapter 30).
4. Keep your cholesterol level below 200 (see Chapter 10).

5. Get a physical exam to check for carotid artery narrowing and signs of heart disease.
6. If you are overweight, get your percent of body fat below 25% (see Chapter 13).
7. If you are diabetic, discuss the hemoglobin A1C blood test with your physician. Ask him or her to use this to help keep the sugar saturation of your red blood cells within desired limits.
8. Check with your health-care provider about the possible advantages of low-dose aspirin therapy in preventing strokes.
9. If you have any symptom that might be a TIA, contact your physician immediately.

Favorite Reading

Stroke: Reducing Your Risk, pamphlet by the National Stroke Association, 300 East Hampden Ave., Suite 240, Englewood, CO 80110-2622; phone 303-762-9922 (publication costs supported by DuPont Pharmaceuticals).

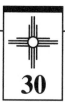

30

BE SMART ABOUT
DRUGS AND ALCOHOL

The most basic suggestions that can be made about drugs are:
1. Don't get started, and,
2. If you already have a problem, get help.

But what do you do about the widespread acceptance of recreational drugs? And what about that common question, "Isn't a drink a day good for you?"

How Dangerous Is Alcohol?

The idea that a drink or two of alcohol each day is "good for you" is controversial. A major study recently reported in the *Harvard Health Letter* claims that alcohol had, at best, only a neutral effect, and was often harmful. Conversely, another large recent study reported in the British journal **Lancet** has found that 1 to 2 drinks a day are protective against heart disease. However, there is a fine line between a drink a day and three drinks a day, a fine line between relaxing and endangering, a fine line between enjoyment and addiction. Three or more alcoholic drinks per day are definitely detrimental to your health.

Questionnaire

How can you tell if you or a friend or a close family member is in danger? The best tool we've seen is an adaptation by Ann Landers of an early questionnaire from the National Council on Alcoholism and Drug Dependence (reproduced with permission). Check off your answers on the left.

Y	N	1. Do you occasionally drink heavily after a disappointment, or a quarrel, or when the boss gives you a hard time?
Y	N	2. When you have trouble or feel under pressure, do you drink more heavily than usual?
Y	N	3. Have you noticed that you are able to handle more liquor than when you first started to drink?
Y	N	4. Did you ever wake up the "morning after" and discover that you could not remember part of the evening before, even though you did not pass out?

Y N	5.	When drinking with others, do you try to sneak extra drinks behind the backs of your companions?
Y N	6.	Are there occasions when you feel uncomfortable if alcohol is not available?
Y N	7.	Have you noticed that you are in more of a hurry to get the first drink than you used to be?
Y N	8.	Do you sometimes feel guilty about your drinking?
Y N	9.	Do you become irritated and defensive when your family or friends bring up the subject of your drinking?
Y N	10.	Have you recently noticed an increase in the frequency of your memory lapses and "blackouts"?
Y N	11.	Do you often wish to continue drinking after your friends say that they have had enough?
Y N	12.	Do you look for reasons to drink heavily, such as the celebration of a big event or after a disappointment or a loss?
Y N	13.	When you are sober, do you regret things you did or said while drinking?
Y N	14.	Have you tried switching brands or following different patterns in an effort to control your drinking?
Y N	15.	Have you failed to keep the promises you made to yourself about cutting down on your drinking?
Y N	16.	Have you ever tried to control your drinking by changing jobs or moving to a new location?
Y N	17.	Do you attempt to avoid family or close friends while you are drinking?
Y N	18.	Are you having an increasing number of financial and work problems?
Y N	19.	Do more people seem to be treating you unfairly without good reason?
Y N	20.	Do you eat very little or skip a meal when you are drinking?
Y N	21.	Do you sometimes have the shakes in the morning and take a drink to "steady your nerves"?
Y N	22.	Have you noticed recently that you cannot drink as much as you once did?
Y N	23.	Do you sometimes stay drunk for several days at a time?
Y N	24.	Do you sometimes feel depressed and wonder whether life is worth living?
Y N	25.	After periods of drinking, do you see or hear things that aren't there?
Y N	26.	Do you become frightened of things you cannot explain after you have been drinking?

If you answered "Yes" to any of the questions, you have some symptoms that may indicate alcoholism. "Yes" answers may indicate the following stages of alcoholism:

"Yes" to questions Numbers 1–8: Early stage
9–21: Middle stage
22–26: Beginning of final stage.

Try this quiz again, replacing "drinking" with "doing drugs."

In 1990 sociologist Lillian Rubin said in *Erotic Wars*, "Yes, crack and cocaine are important, but alcohol is what parents in this country ought to be most concerned about." *Erotic Wars* is based on interviews of nearly 1,000 students and young adults in the U.S., and her estimate is that "fully 10% of the college-campus students were on their way to becoming alcoholics." Similar warnings about the dangers of alcohol have come from former First Lady Betty Ford and Kitty Dukakis.

As the U.S. Dept. of Transportation and The Advertising Council, Inc., remind us, "Friends don't let friends drive drunk."

Some Facts about Drinking and Drugs

- Driving after drinking causes 23,000 deaths every year, which is nearly half of all automobile fatalities.
- Alcohol causes more than 15% of all deaths in this country every year.
- One-fourth of Americans in hospitals have alcohol-related problems.
- 40 states use sobriety roadblocks.
- 10% of Americans use illicit drugs at least once a month: 4 to 5 million use cocaine; 20 million use marijuana; 20 million use prescription drugs for non-medical reasons.
- There are 3,000 cocaine-related deaths each year in this country.
- Drugs cost us over $177 billion each year in missed work, health care, and crime.
- In nearly 20% of all divorces, alcohol abuse by a spouse is cited as a significant cause.

Recommendations

1. If you like beer, experiment with some of the excellent non-alcoholic alternatives, such as Clausthaler, Norsk, Kaliber, O'Doul's, Sharp's, Wartech, Haake-Beck, Firestone, and Buckler.
2. Try Ariel Winery's variety of de-alcoholized wines, especially their champagne (Napa, California; 800-456-9472).
3. If you like wine with dinner, but don't want to feel like you have to "finish off" the whole bottle, buy a nitrogen canister from Private Preserve (707-252-4258).
4. Try Martinelli's non-alcoholic sparkling cider.
5. If you like good wine, buy a bottle of Opus One; you won't have any money left over to overdo the cheap stuff.
6. Give the questionnaire in this chapter to a friend.
7. Serve as a designated driver for someone who has been drinking.
8. If you have any symptoms of addiction to drugs or alcohol, contact Narcotics Anonymous or Alcoholics Anonymous. The "Twelve-Step" groups are free, and they work. They are the original peer-counseling support networks.

Recommended Resources

For general information and support groups:

Alcoholics Anonymous: Check your local telephone directory, or write to Alcoholics Anonymous, GSO, Box 459, Grand Central Station, NY 10017.

Al-Anon/Alateen for the families and friends of alcoholics, 212-302-7240.

Narcotics Anonymous: Check your local telephone directory or call 818-780-3951.

National Council on Alcoholism and Drug Dependence, 800-622-2255.

"Just Say No" Foundation, Walnut Creek, CA, 800-258-2766, or 510-939-6666 locally.

If you wish to assist high-school students with alcohol restraint, call SADD (Students Against Driving Drunk) 508-481-3568.

If you're interested in a political action group, contact MADD (Mothers Against Drunk Driving) 800-438-6233. Ask about their guide "Operation Prom Graduation" as to how to safely celebrate high-school graduation.

Women for Sobriety, a national self-help program for women, 215-536-8026.

If you have an immediate problem or question, use these

24-HOUR HOTLINE NUMBERS:

Alcohol, 800-ALCALLS

Al-Anon/Alateen, 800-356-9996

Cocaine, 800-COCAINE

Pride-Drug Education, 800-677-7433

National Criminal Justice, 800-GIVE-TIP.

Favorite Readings

Alcoholism: How to Recognize It, How to Deal With It, How to Conquer It, and *The Lowdown on Dope*, both by Ann Landers, Box 11562, Chicago, IL 60611.

Keep Off the Grass and *Cocaine: The Great White Plague*, by Gabriel Nahas, M.D., Middlebury, VT: Paul S. Ericksson Publishing Co., 1985, 304 pgs.

Marijuana: Myths and Misconceptions, by Robert C. Gilkeson, M.D., The Center for Drug Education and Brain Research, Cos Cob, CT 06807.

31

STOP SMOKING

"You can spend $64 on a stop-smoking class or $100,000 on a lifetime of smoking," said former Surgeon General Dr. Everett Koop. That may be oversimplifying things, but the costs of smoking to both your health and your finances can be considerable.

Stopping smoking isn't easy. Nicotine can be as addictive as heroin. And many former smokers have quit repeatedly before finally succeeding. In spite of the difficulties, four thousand adults successfully give up smoking *every day* in the U.S.! As columnist George Will reflected, "20 years from now the ashtray may have gone the way of the spittoon."

Some Facts about Smoking

- Cigarette smoking is the number-one cause of preventable death in this country.
- If you're a 30-year-old smoker, you can expect to live 18 years *less* than your nonsmoking peer; if you're 60 and smoking, subtract 11 years from your life expectancy.
- Smokers have a higher incidence of throat cancer, breast cancer, lung cancer, bladder cancer, heart attacks, emphysema, osteoporosis, strokes, and several other diseases than do nonsmokers.
- A smoker's increased risk of dying from a heart attack largely disappears within two to three years of quitting smoking.
- The single largest cause of low-birthweight babies in this country is mothers who smoke cigarettes during pregnancy.
- Children's respiratory infections (colds, croup, bronchitis, pneumonia) will last a third *longer* if they live with a smoker.
- If either parent smokes, the odds are 50-50 that their children will grow up to be smokers.
- Surgeon General Dr. Antonia Novello reported in 1990 that more than *three thousand* teenagers in the U.S. become addicted to smoking *every day*.

Weight Gain and Smoking Cessation

Gaining weight is a realistic concern among smokers about to quit. Recent studies have shown that, on average, a former smoker will gain 6 to 8 pounds upon quitting. However, to offset the tremendous health benefits of smoking cessation, a person would have to gain more than 85 pounds. The key advice in this area is to take up a regular physical activity at the same time you give up smoking.

Risk of Mouth and Throat Cancer

Many Americans don't realize that Babe Ruth, after chewing tobacco for many years during his baseball career, died of throat cancer at age 52. Dr. Bobby Brown, president of the American League, has banned chewing tobacco at the ball park as of spring 1991 by all minor-league players and coaches. Ear, nose, and throat specialist Dr. Roy Sessions was quoted by the *AMA News* as saying, in reference to switching from smoking tobacco to chewing tobacco, "You're just trading lung cancer for mouth cancer" (30,000 new cases in the U.S. per year).

Recommendations

1. Quit smoking!
2. If you must smoke, and you live with others, smoke somewhere else (on your porch, in your car, in your own office, outdoors).
3. If you are pregnant and must smoke, cut down to six or fewer cigarettes per day.
4. If you've quit before, and restarted, join a quit-smoking class at work or through your health-care provider. Pick a date to quit. For example, you might try the "The Great American Smoke Out," which is a day in November when smokers are urged to quit smoking for that day. Make an action plan for quitting and be sure to identify supportive people to help you succeed. Buy dozens of packs of sugarless chewing gum or a can of cinnamon spice sticks. Start a new physical activity, such as jogging, bicycling, or swimming, at the same time to reinforce your body's independence from cigarettes.

Favorite Reading

The American Cancer Society's *Fresh Start: 21 Days to Stop Smoking*, by Dee Burton, Ph.D. New York: Pocket Books, 1986, 159 pgs.

Answer:
Three thousand

32

AVOID PASSIVE SMOKE

Many people know that smoking cigarettes is the number-one cause of preventable, disease-related deaths in this country. Alcohol abuse ranks number two. But did you know that passive cigarette smoke — from other people's cigarettes — is number three?

How Dangerous Is Passive Smoke?

In 1986 the U.S. Surgeon General announced that nonsmokers exposed to passive smoke are at increased risk of dying from lung cancer. In June 1990 the Environmental Protection Agency released its long-awaited report declaring environmental tobacco smoke a "known human carcinogen." In the U.S., this translates into nearly 4,000 unexpected lung-cancer deaths each year! Added to this number are several thousand unexpected "miscellaneous" cancer deaths related to other people's cigarette smoke, bladder cancer and pancreatic cancer among them.

The gasses from cigarette smoke (carbon monoxide, nitrous oxide, nicotine, ammonia, nitrosamine) are *more* concentrated in environmental smoke, or "sidestream smoke," than they are in the smoke that the smoker inhales! When a smoker inhales and draws in oxygen, some of these gasses are diluted; if the cigarette is filtered, even more substances are removed. A nearby nonsmoker is not protected by either of these two processes.

"Nonsmokers who live with smokers have a 20 to 30% higher risk of dying from heart disease than do other nonsmokers," says Dr. Stanton Glantz, of U.C. Medical Center at San Francisco (see *Circulation*, January 1991 issue). This means that if your spouse smokes and you don't, *you* are still at risk for heart disease! Second-hand cigarette smoke results in 32,000 excess heart-disease deaths in this country every year.

Deaths from Passive Smoking

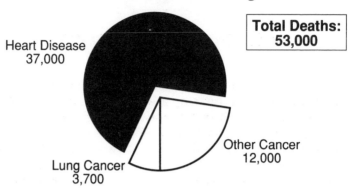

Heart Disease
37,000

**Total Deaths:
53,000**

Other Cancer
12,000

Lung Cancer
3,700

Reproduced with permission of Dr. Stanton Glantz, A. Judson Wells, Ph.D., and the American Heart Association, Inc.

Effects on Children

Other recent medical reports of note include a National Cancer Institute report that a child growing up with two parents who smoke has twice the risk of dying in later life from lung cancer (*New England Journal of Medicine*, Sept. 1990). Both leukemia and brain cancer are increased in children whose father smoked (*American Journal of Epidemiology*, Jan. 1991). Pneumonia, asthma, and persistent ear infections are all related to maternal cigarette smoking.

Recommendations

1. If you can, avoid public places where smoking is allowed. Request nonsmoking seating in restaurants and airplanes.
2. Request (insist) that if people around you must smoke, they smoke outside.

Favorite Reading

Facts about Second-Hand Smoke, by the American Lung Association, 1740 Broadway, New York, NY 10019; 212- 315-8700; free with a self-addressed stamped envelope.

Answer:
500 billion

33

REDUCE YOUR STRESS

Stress is not necessarily bad. Public speakers, executives, students, and others commonly refer to "good stress" as that impetus which helps them deliver a better performance, finish an assignment, meet a deadline, etc. But if you took a poll of your friends or colleagues, a majority would likely respond that they have "too much stress" in their lives. High levels of stress have been found to be correlated with an increased risk of heart attacks and strokes, and a weakened immune system. The following suggestions from friends and various health journals may help you lower excess stress in your life.

Recommendations

1. Try whistling or humming at work.
2. Beware of bosses who scream.
3. "Learn how to juggle colorful scarves as a stress-reducing technique; and every once in a while, let one fall to the floor, to learn how to deal with failure." Steve Allen, Jr., M.D.
4. Take a trip by train instead of driving.
5. To learn how to be calmer in traffic, read *Drive With Less Stress* by Dr. Lesser (Los Angeles, CA: Less Stress Press, 1989).
6. Go on a cruise.
7. Take a vacation for a week — with no TV.
8. Learn T'ai chi, transcendental meditation, or yoga.
9. Consider singer and author Holly Near's insight, "The change came when I realized that you don't have to do it all yourself in the next 10 minutes."
10. Don't go to bed angry. Competitive, hard-driving people *with suppressed anger and rage* endanger their health more than any other group.
11. Switch from caffeinated to decaffeinated beverages.
12. Find quiet alone time each day.

13. "Eliminate the clutter from your life" (*East West Journal*, May 1991).
14. Have a massage.
15. Treat yourself to cut flowers.

Recommended Resource

Pelican Tape Series by Phyllis Ward, 3731 S. Glenstone #90, Springfield, MO 65804, especially "Basic Relaxation" and "As You Like It"

Favorite Readings

Kicking Your Stress Habits, Donald Tubesing, Whole Person Associates, Inc., 1702 E. Jefferson, Duluth, MN 55812; 218-728-6807, 189 pgs.

The 14-Day Stress Cure: A New Approach for Dealing with Stress That Can Change Your Life, Mort Orman, M.D. Houston, TX: Breakthru Publishing, 1991; 800-227-1152; 348 pgs.

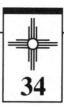

34

MAINTAIN YOUR FRIENDSHIPS

Isolated people don't live as long. Many of us have known or heard of someone who has died shortly after the death of their spouse. They seem to have just given up "the will to live." But it has to do with more than simply grieving. When dealing with isolation, divorced and never-married adults are especially vulnerable. This is becoming even more important as Americans who are now 65 can expect, on average, to live into their 80s.

What Are the Benefits of Friendship?

In his workshop *Self-Care for the Busy Professional*, medical anthropologist John-Henry Pfifferling, Ph.D., spends much time on the importance of protecting and nurturing relationships. He asks, "Do you have a love relationship?" and "Do you have someone with whom you can discuss your problems, needs, and successes?" Unfortunately, some people get so busy that their relationships are one of the first things to be squeezed out when there's not enough time to go around.

Those in successful marriages will usually agree that they've had to work on their marriage; they've worked at maintaining communication, being open to compromises, and remaining sensitive. Friendships require work as well. If you don't put enough effort into maintaining a regular connection, it will gradually diminish.

It has been said that women have many close friends, but that men basically have their wives. Perhaps this is not as true today, when so many women are struggling to balance roles as wage-earners, mothers, wives, and household managers. For women as well as for men, friendships can easily be a casualty of a busy life. But, in general, men in our culture have a more limited network of close friends and have the most to gain by taking the time to maintain their friendships.

In her insightful book *Just Friends,* sociologist Lillian Rubin explains the various roles and various types of friends in our lives. She describes "special friends who have shared the mundane details of everyday living along with the extraordinary events," new friends and old friends, friends who are "like a brother" or "just like a sister," "playmates" and "soulmates," "friends of the road" and "friends of the heart," "special purpose" friends, opposite-sex friends, "just friends," good friends, and "best" friends. All are important in their own way. "Our friends ease the shifts and changes we experience as we live through the various life stages."

Recommendations

1. Sometime in the coming month, schedule lunch or dinner with a nearly lost friend.
2. Schedule regular time with at least two valued friends outside of your primary relationship.
3. Call your friends or send them a hand-written note when you know something significant has happened in their lives (they've given a presentation, gotten the results of lab tests from their doctor, returned from a trip, etc.).
4. Look up former friends from school or your childhood neighborhood.
5. Learn to develop your friendships in ways that are not competitive.
6. Build and maintain a variety of friendships to sustain and enrich your later years. It's especially important to have good friends after retirement and after the death of your spouse.

Favorite Reading

Just Friends: The Role of Friendship in Our Lives, by Lillian B. Rubin. New York: Harper & Row, 1985, 235 pgs.

Answer:

80 for men, 84 for women

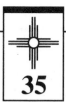

35

GET A PET

Two men each had a heart attack one year ago. One of them has a pet dog; the other doesn't. The one who has the pet is statistically the one more likely to be alive today.

What Are the Benefits of Owning a Pet?

The benefits of a pet involve more than the fact that their owners might get more exercise walking their animal. For elderly adults in a nursing home, or for cancer patients on a hospice ward, a pet provides hours of companionship. For children, a pet provides unconditional love. Psychologically withdrawn or mentally impaired children derive benefit especially from larger animals such as cows. Studies have shown that prisoners learn compassion from pets. Other studies show that adults who have high blood pressure will have their blood pressure lowered by watching a fish tank, or petting a dog or cat. Severely paralyzed or blind individuals in this country commonly rely on trained animals to perform all sorts of everyday tasks. And for persons with AIDS and other serious diseases, a pet can provide a reason for living.

The health benefits a pet provides apply whether you live in your own home or in an institution. Nearly 25 medical studies have shown that the presence of pets will result in more smiling, more conversation, greater reaching out to others, less agitation, more alertness, and less depression.

Time spent with a cat on your lap can never be considered totally wasted.

Recommendation

Consider whether a pet might add companionship and enjoyment to your or your family's life, provided you have the time and energy to be a responsible pet owner.

Recommended Resources

For information on senior citizens (over 60) adopting pets at a reduced cost through the Purina Pets for People Program, contact the Animal Protective League, 1729 Willey Ave., Cleveland, OH 44113; 216-771-4616.

Favorite Reading

For a resource list of pet-related books, medical references, posters, and audiovisuals, write to the Delta Society, Box 1080, Renton, WA 98057-1080; 206-226-7357.

Answer:
Cats (66,000,000 compared to 45,000,000 dogs)

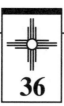

36

PROTECT YOUR ENVIRONMENT

If it is true that "We are what we eat," then perhaps it's also true that "We are what we drink" and "We are what we breathe." Society as a whole is becoming more environmentally aware, and with good reason: there are pesticides in the ground and water, pollutants in our air above, and radon leaking up from below. Pollution can not only damage our health physically, but also erode our morale and our will to live.

Our environment directly affects our health. In Oregon, the Lane County Medical Society used Earth Day 1990 to promote its energy conservation and recycling efforts. A few of their measures include: using only recycled paper, canceling unnecessary subscriptions, and recycling plastic. Society president John Allcott, M.D., explains, "What's good for the environment is also good for people."

Recommendations

1. Stop junk mail.
2. Get people at work involved with you in an "Environmental Task Force."
3. Recycle your family's aluminum cans, glass, newspapers, and plastic.
4. Get your office cafeteria or favorite café to offer a 5- cent discount to those who bring their own mug instead of using a throw-away cup.
5. Learn how to start a compost pile, and add worms.
6. Sort and recycle white paper, colored paper, glossy paper, and cardboard at work.
7. If you live in a home with older plumbing, have your drinking water tested for excessive lead. Check with your water-supply district.

8. If your community doesn't have a curbside recycling program, find out how to start one.
9. For diabetics and others who use needles, lancets, or other sharp objects, dispose of these carefully in a hard-plastic or metal container with a secure lid.
10. Check with your local health department to see whether or not your house and basement are located in a high radon area.
11. Buy a copy of *50 Simple Things Kids Can Do to Save the Earth* and give it to a child or teenager.
12. Carpool to work at least once a week.
13. Subscribe to one of the many ecology periodicals.
14. Precycle, that is, reuse rather than purchase another.

Recommended Resource

An excellent ecology journal is the monthly *Green Consumer Letter*, 1526 Connecticut Ave. NW, Washington, DC 20036; 800-955-4733.

Favorite Reading

50 Simple Things You Can Do to Save the Earth, Berkeley, CA: The EarthWorks Group, 1989, 96 pgs.

37

HONOR YOUR PERSONAL TRADITIONS

"To a child, once is a tradition." So said author Dolores Curran at a parenting workshop several years ago. She told the story a mother had shared with her about having introduced her children to the custom of dying Easter eggs one spring. The next year this mother decided to buy colored decals for her children to decorate the eggs with. To her dismay, her children were not pleased with her switch. "But Mom," they protested, "we *always* dye our eggs!"

Why Are Traditions Important?

Ms. Curran, a former schoolteacher from Denver, Colorado, sent out 500 surveys to school principals, counselors, ministers, pediatricians, and others, asking the question, "What qualities do healthy families possess?" To her surprise she received more than 550 surveys back! People were so intrigued by her project that they copied her survey and shared it with colleagues. Their responses helped create her book, *Traits of A Healthy Family*, which won the Christopher Book Award in 1983. This is the best book we have found on what is *right* with American families; Chapter 8 of her book deals with the value of family rituals and traditions.

We have a friend who used to be given raspberry sherbet, in addition to tea and crackers, when recovering from the usual childhood illnesses. Today, 30 years later, he still buys himself raspberry sherbet to nurse himself through colds and the flu. Some families rely on chicken soup. In some pediatric clinics today, rainbow sherbet has become the "tradition" of choice. And thousands of kids count on getting ice cream as a reward for going through tonsil surgery.

There is an abundance of ritual and tradition used by American families. Many family rituals are intended to help us coordinate our family schedules, to organize our lives, and to prepare the family for the outside world.

Traditions provide a sense of continuity with our own immediate family's past, as well as that of all humanity. "Tradition reaches like a lifeline across the generations," wrote novelist John Dos Passos. It also provides a sense of continuity with our collective future.

Your Family's Traditions

Check off the rituals and traditions in this list that you and your family share:

- [ ] Thanksgiving dinner with family members
- [ ] Christmas lists for Santa Claus
- [ ] Hanukkah
- [ ] Fourth of July fireworks and neighborhood barbecues
- [ ] Graduation ceremonies
- [ ] Bar Mitzvah and Bat Mitzvah
- [ ] Baptism/First Communion/Confirmation
- [ ] Shopping for a new notebook, crayons, and pencils for the first day of school
- [ ] Children mowing the lawn
- [ ] Evening walks with the family dog
- [ ] Wedding vows, toasts, and honeymoons
- [ ] Saving a lost tooth for the tooth fairy
- [ ] Staying out late the night of your senior prom (even if you're having a terrible time)
- [ ] Putting flowers on a loved one's grave
- [ ] Passover Seders
- [ ] Super Bowl parties
- [ ] Family dinners around the dining-room table
- [ ] Celebrating birthdays and anniversaries
- [ ] Sending valentines to loved ones
- [ ] Class rings
- [ ] Wearing a Halloween costume, carving pumpkins, "Trick or Treating"
- [ ] Baby showers
- [ ] Meeting a friend for coffee

☐ Celebrating the swallows' return to Capistrano, the butterflies' gathering in Pacific Grove, or, whatever your local tradition might be

☐ Having grandparents retell the family stories.

Recommendations

1. Think twice before you discard a "silly" family tradition.
2. If you don't have an annual event at which family members or friends gather, choose one, and invite them.
3. For young adults forming families, give thought to creating your own traditions as well as including some of those you grew up with.

Favorite Reading

Traits of A Healthy Family, by Dolores Curran. New York: Ballantine, 1983, 322 pgs.

38

DEVELOP YOUR HOBBY

At the end of a workshop on hobbies and health promotion, librarian Alice Wygant of Galveston, Texas, volunteered that her hobby is collecting porcelain plates in the shape of strawberries. Others have suggested hobbies such as collecting baseball hats, making stained-glass windows, seeking out the perfect swimming hole, collecting memorable stones, operating an amateur radio, painting miniature figures, growing a variety of palm trees, flower arranging, bird watching, or playing any one of a variety of musical instruments. The main requirement for any hobby is that it be *important* to you.

What Are the Health Benefits of Hobbies?

Hawaiian physician John Dillon, of Koloa, Kauai, recently provided a useful definition of a hobby: "An activity or interest done for pleasure or relaxation and not as a main occupation." A hobby can energize a person, when one feels otherwise drained. Dr. Dillon finishes his advice by saying, "It is never too late to start, but now is better." Another successful leader, Texas manager Ed Platt, was recently quoted, "I now do energizing hobbies during the time after work that I used to spend just being tired."

Stress-management consultant Phyllis Ward of Springfield, Missouri, used to feel that she couldn't tell a joke. To get through a difficult time in her life, she decided to learn one new joke every week. She would practice these "groaners" on her office-mates, and found that she gradually lost her self-consciousness about telling jokes. Soon she was learning a new joke every day, and now says, "I guess it's become a sort of hobby." Her new hobby provided both healing and personal growth.

When does a hobby become an addiction?

In an insightful workshop called *Self-Care For The Busy Professional*, John-Henry Pfifferling of Durham, North Carolina, claims that hobbies are not only important and legitimate, but essential for a well-balanced life. He suggests that if you have an occupation, for example, as a counselor or therapist, in which successes or resolutions can take months to evolve, that you take up a finite hobby, for example, completing jigsaw puzzles or painting miniature figurines, from which you get more immediate validation and sense of completion.

Recommendations

1. Ask yourself, "What in your life gives you pleasure and relaxes you?"
2. Make sure you set aside time each week to be involved in these activities.
3. If you don't have any current hobbies or ideas, draw on favorite childhood pastimes.

Favorite Reading

Society for Professional Well-Being quarterly newsletter, 21 West Colony Place #150, Durham, NC 27705.

Answer:
When it controls you

39

LIGHTEN UP

Why are we oftentimes so hard on ourselves? Have you ever spent time listening to your own "self talk"? It can be depressing. As health specialists David Sobel and Robert Ornstein said in *Healthy Pleasures*, "Most of us don't take laughter seriously enough."

How Therapeutic Is a Light-Hearted Attitude?

On the first evening of a wellness conference in Philadelphia, in April 1990, the participants were asked to introduce themselves to the stranger next to them, and then vividly tell in one minute the three worst things that had happened to them in the previous 24 hours. For example, "My cab was held up in traffic and I missed my original flight; one of my suitcases is still missing; and I've only had four hours sleep." Then they switched, so the other person could tell their story. The next step was to describe with equal drama the same three events and *what was so wonderful* about them. For example, "I missed my flight, which gave me an extra three hours to read the novel I've been carrying around with me for six months; I lost my suitcase, so I went out and bought myself my first new suit in two years; and I discovered I'm functioning better on four hours sleep than I ever thought I could!" You could almost palpate the change in the atmosphere in the room. Ask yourself how, by focusing on the bright side of a recent event in your life, you could reframe a negative experience as a positive or growthful one.

In addition to the mental-health benefits of focusing on the positive, a light-hearted attitude can have physical benefits as well. Vigorous laughter produces a brief workout for your heart, and exercise for your abdominal and diaphragm muscles. As the laughter subsides, your body relaxes. Some people claim that frequent laughter actually decreases their craving for unnecessary snacks.

Author Norman Cousins once described laughter as "a form of jogging for the innards." In his book *Anatomy of an Illness*, he eloquently tells how his recovery from a mysterious,

Who said, "Half of the game is 90 percent mental."?

life-threatening illness was partly due to watching reruns of *Candid Camera* television shows. When his rare illness was diagnosed, and his physician told him that his chances for recovery were about 1 in 100, he decided to take the management of his own case largely into his own hands. "I can do better than that," he figured. So he checked out of his hospital bed and into a hotel ("Whoever gets a good night's sleep in a hospital?"). He also hired private nurses to regulate his medications, took vitamin C daily, ate wisely, and spent an hour a day laughing at *Candid Camera* reruns. He gradually recovered. Subsequently, he stressed the value of "positive" emotions such as festivity, love, faith, sense of purpose, and a strong will to live.

Recommendations

1. Pay attention to taking yourself less seriously.
2. Learn to notice when you are being judgmental *of others*.
3. Learn to see and laugh at your own shortcomings.
4. Ask yourself if anyone else will remember in a year the fool you thought you made of yourself today.
5. Rent a copy of Bill Cosby's comedy video.
6. Go to a magic or novelty shop, and give yourself permission to buy something that appeals to your playful side.
7. Watch an episode on television of "America's Funniest Home Videos."
8. Develop friendships with optimists, and spend less time with people who are pessimists.
9. Send for Steve Allen, Jr., M.D.'s video *Juggling Life's Stress*, available from M.D. Enterprises, 8 La Grand Court, Ithaca, NY 14850; 607-277-1795.
10. Subscribe to the *Humor Perspective* newsletter, available from Ruth Hamilton, Carolina Health and Humor Association, 5223 Revere Road, Durham, NC 27713.
11. Remind yourself of that obscure quote by Sebastian Roch Nicolas Chamfort, "The most utterly lost of all days is that in which we have not once laughed."

Favorite Reading

Healthy Pleasures, by David Sobel, M.D., and Robert Ornstein, Ph.D. Reading, MA: Addison-Wesley, 1989, 302 pgs.

Answer:
Baseball-manager Yogi Berra

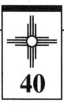

40

LOVE YOUR JOB,
OR FIND ONE YOU CAN LOVE

A medical colleague recently confided that he used to go to work regularly with stomach pains and a headache. He said that by the time he came home, both would be worse. He then joined another medical clinic. "The day I made the decision to change jobs, the stomachaches went away. The day I left my old job, the headaches went away."

How Does Our Job Affect Our Health?

How much we enjoy our work (or dislike it) directly affects how we feel about ourselves and how we feel in general. Physicians who take care of adults know that asking, "Do you like your work?" often gives them the best indication of that person's state of general health. People who answer "No" are more likely to have back trouble, headaches, abdominal difficulties, and high blood pressure, and will use more sick days off from work than those who can answer "Yes."

Psychologist Abraham Maslow went so far as to say, "The only happy people I know are the ones who are working well at something they consider important." Dennis Jaffe and Cynthia Scott in their book *Take This Job and Love It* said, "Working only so that you can enjoy your time off is perhaps the greatest threat to your health and well-being." And Managing Editor of the *Wall Street Journal* Norman Pearlstine pointed to "a passion for one's work" as a common trait among today's successful executives.

Another factor affecting our satisfaction with our work is the rate of change in today's workplace. Author Tom Peters, in his books *Thriving on Chaos* and *In Search of Excellence,* points out that within the space of a year or two we are now having to adapt to changes that used to take decades. Peters advocates acknowledging and welcoming such challenges. The most successful individuals and companies will be those who not only tolerate change, but actually thrive on it.

Recommendations

1. Decide for yourself how to use your work to boost your self-esteem and raise the level of personal satisfaction in your life.
2. To better understand your personality traits and job fit, send for a copy of Wenham's CEO profile (5755 Granger Rd. #400, Independence, OH 44131).
3. Consider whether you should be in another type of work that you would enjoy more. To begin such a consideration, read Richard Bolles' best-selling *What Color Is Your Parachute?*

Favorite Readings

Take This Job and Love It, by Dennis Jaffe, Ph.D. and Cynthia Scott, Ph.D. New York: Simon and Schuster, 1988, 219 pgs.

The Way of the Ronin: Riding the Waves of Change at Work, by Beverly Potter, Ph.D. Berkeley, CA: Ronin Publishers, 1984, 243 pgs.

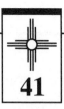

41

AFFIRM YOURSELF

In May 1991 a study appeared linking perfectionism to anxiety disorders. People with high degrees of stubbornness, repressed emotions, indecision, excessive devotion to work, and unrealistic self-expectations seem to be the ones at most risk for a variety of anxiety-related problems.

According to interviews and ratings used by Dr. Gerald Nestadt at Baltimore's Johns Hopkins School of Medicine, these traits were found to be present in urban U.S. residents to the degrees shown in the table. Learning the art of self-affirmation is one of the most effective tools you can use to overcome these character traits.

Percentage of People with These Traits

	Moderate degree	Severe degree
Perfectionism	31%	8%
Stubbornness	28%	12%
Indecision	9%	2%
Excessive work devotion	14%	4%
Emotional constriction	16%	4%

Popular therapist David Burns, M.D., in his best-selling *Feeling Good,* says "you feel the way you think. Only your own sense of self-worth determines how you feel." In response to the question, "Then how can I develop a sense of self-esteem?" he answers, "You don't have to! . . . all you have to do is turn off that critical, haranguing, inner voice." In his book he explains the basic technique of countering or rebutting in writing every negative or self-critical thought you might have by writing down a rational response.

Which famous American said, "Those things that hurt, instruct."?

Perhaps the best book devoted to the skill of positive self-talk is Pamela Butler's *Talking To Yourself: Learning the Language of Self-Support*. The book begins, "We all talk to ourselves." She goes on to give examples of internal dialogues and of how to convert draining judgments about ourselves into positive affirmations. In particular she discusses common roadblocks, such as shoulds and should nots, overly rigid standards, negative self-labeling, and catastrophizing. Common self-defeating refrains include "Hurry up," "What if?" "Don't be different," "That's stupid," and "No time for . . ." Learning to avoid these traps can be liberating and growthful.

Recommendations

1. Learn the skill of self-affirmation.
2. On your drive home from work, tell yourself what positive accomplishments you've achieved that day.
3. Find out what classes are offered through your community or place of work on stress reduction and other coping techniques.
4. Be easier on yourself.
5. "Set attainable goals" (Zen saying).

Favorite Reading

Talking to Yourself: Learning the Language of Self-Support, by Pamela Butler, Ph.D. San Francisco: Harper and Row, 1981, 204 pgs.

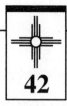

42

VISUALIZE YOUR GOALS

One night at the dinner table, a 44-year-old woman announced to her family that she was going back to college. "But, Mom," one of her sons protested, "you'll be 48 when you graduate!"

"I'll be 48 anyway," was her reply.

Select Your Goals Carefully

Before graduation, some students of the Harvard Business School complete an exercise describing where they would like to be in five years: what field they see themselves in, what position they will hold in that field, etc. The instructions are followed by this warning, "Be careful in the goals you set for yourself, because you will probably achieve them." Admittedly, we don't all have the skills and privileges that go along with an education at Harvard Business School, but the lesson for each of us remains the same.

Setting a goal and achieving that goal is one of life's most satisfying experiences. Norman Vincent Peale lectured extensively on the value of goal setting and positive thinking, and his book *The Power of Positive Thinking* has sold more than 3 million copies. Goal-setting and the process used in doing so varies tremendously from person to person. Some people are most creative early in the morning; others are "afternoon people" or "night people." Many business people use commute time, either on the highway or in a plane, to gain perspective. Others go on weekend retreats. One friend uses her birthday to go to a hilltop and reexamine her life.

As writer Robert Greenleaf said, "Nothing much happens without a dream."

What percent of Americans have clearly thought-out goals and have written them down?

Recommendations

1. Leave the car radio off during part of your driving time; it's a good time to be alone with your thoughts and feelings.
2. Each month, find a fresh person or a book that is unrelated to your work, to help expand your usual horizons.
3. Divide your goals for the year into monthly, quarterly, or seasonal goals; this makes them appear more achievable, and makes any shortfalls during the year seem less defeating.
4. Be sure to write your goals down.
5. Heed Joseph Campbell's advice, "Follow your bliss."
6. Choose your goals carefully; you're apt to achieve them.

Favorite Readings

Creative Visualization, by Shakti Gawain. San Rafael, CA: New World Library, 1978, 158 pgs.

Empowerment: The Art of Creating Your Life As You Want It, by David Gershon and Gail Straub. New York: Delta, 1989, 235 pgs.

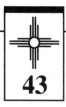

43

USE YOUR UNCONSCIOUS

When a group of prominent thinkers and historians were asked what they thought was the most significant development of the 20th century, they gave an answer which might surprise you. They might have answered Einstein's theory of relativity, the nuclear bomb, or mankind's landing a man on the Moon. Instead, they answered the discovery of the human unconscious. The awareness that many of our actions are subtly, and not so subtly, influenced by forces not immediately accessible to our consciousness is of tremendous significance as we head into the 21st century.

How Much of Your Unconscious Do You Tap Into?

How many times have you made the same mistake over and over? Or made "Freudian slips" in your conversation? Or pursued a course of action you knew to be "irrational"? Sometimes we do well to follow our instincts. At other times we find ourselves in a rut, pursuing goals of questionable value for unclear reasons.

Parents may be able to recognize their unconscious coming to the surface when they surprise themselves by parenting in a certain way, and exclaiming to themselves, "That's just like my mother (or father)." Therapist and currently popular author John Bradshaw writes of the 29,000 hours of programming we have experienced in our childhoods. Whether for better or for worse, our responses as parents to various situations seem to arise "automatically." It requires great conscious attention to change these patterns.

The richest source of information about our own unique unconscious is provided by our dreams. Sigmund Freud at the turn of the century termed dreams "the royal road to the unconscious." All of us dream, but not all of us remember our dreams. Some of us are fortunate enough to dream in color. Dreams can be recalled with some practice.

The second great revolutionary thinker in this field was Swiss psychiatrist Carl Jung, who published more than twenty volumes of his life's work. His autobiography, *Memories, Dreams, Reflections,*

What percent of adults report that they dream in their sleep?

written at age 83, begins, "My life is a story of the self-realization of the unconscious." And later, "The story of a life begins somewhere, at some particular point we happen to remember; and even then it was already highly complex." For himself he says, "I early arrived at the insight that when no answer comes from within to the problems and complexities of life, they ultimately mean very little." Jung used retreats into his study, his painting, hewing stones, and his dreams to give him guidance in life.

Author Norman Cousin's account (*This Train Doesn't Stop in Baltimore*) of a dream he had while in a hospital is one of the most moving ever published. In the middle of the night, fearing his life was nearing its end, he awoke in a cold sweat on the floor of his hospital room. He had dreamt of a heavy old train ("Death") slowing to a halt at a symbolic train station. He found himself sprawled in his hospital gown amidst his IV tubing screaming, "This train doesn't stop in Baltimore." He resolved that he was not yet ready to die. And he recovered.

Psychiatrist Keith Harary, M.D., author of *Lucid Dreams in 30 Days*, has said, "I think if you really got into lucid dreaming on a deep and ongoing basis, you are bound to develop a more expansive view of yourself, your potential, and everyday reality."

Recommendations

1. Consider buying a book in which to record your dreams. Record them in the present tense (in writing or by tape).
2. Sleep in occasionally, with the expectation of remembering your dreams.
3. Don't wake up to the morning news (or even music) if you wish to hang on to your last dream.
4. Give each of your dreams a title when you write them down. The choice of a title may itself be illuminating.
5. Pay attention to your Freudian slips.
6. Utilize avenues such as painting, clay, sculpting, and journal writing.
7. Share your dreams with those who are close to you, and ask them about their dreams.

Favorite Readings

Dream Work, by Jeremy Taylor. Mahwah, NJ: Paulist Press, 1983, 280 pgs.

The Wisdom of the Dream, by Stephen Segaller and Merrill Berger. Boston: Shambhala Publications, 1989, 211 pgs.

Answer:
65% of men and 71% of women (*Great Divide*, 1991)

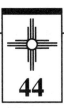

44

SEARCH FOR MEANING

An English couple received a lot of attention a few years ago after winning the lottery, selling their sporting-goods store, and sailing around the world. They received even more attention when they returned after a year, bought another sporting-goods store, and went back to work. "We didn't have any purpose in life," they explained.

Why Is Meaning Important?

The search for meaning in our lives remains a crucial issue. Many use religion to find their meaning. People devote their lives to God, Christ, Buddha, Allah, the Goddess, or a Higher Being, and find their lives enriched. As minister Hank Anderson advises, "Know your God."

Joseph Campbell framed it by saying, "I think that what we're seeking is an experience of being alive . . . so that we actually feel the rapture of being alive." This rapture must have been present for the "Six Across Antarctica" in their heroic quest to be the first non-mechanized expedition to cross the South Pole, as reported in the *National Geographic*. The group included an American science teacher, a French sports-medicine specialist, a Soviet meteorologist, a Chinese geologist, a Japanese sled-dog trainer, and a British navigator. They travelled more than 3,700 miles, and all survived.

Dr. Donald Chung had made a promise to his North Korean mother to return home in three days, but during that interval was drafted into the South Korean army. After 40 years, he was able to return to the site of her grave. From the sales of his book, *The Three-Day Promise*, hè has donated more than $430,000 toward the Korean War Veterans Memorial (scheduled to be dedicated in July of 1993), and his life and work have taken on new meaning for him.

How many high-school seniors say it is important to find purpose and meaning in their lives?

A large percentage of those suffering from depression seem to lack meaning in their lives. Nietzsche has said, "He who has a *why* to live can bear with almost any *how*." From this philosophy and the lifelong work of Viktor Frankl has emerged that special branch of psychology called logotherapy, which seeks to help individuals find meaning in their lives. Dr. Frankl's prescription: "Live as if you were living for the second time and had acted as wrongly the first time as you are about to act now."

The book *The Road Less Traveled* seems to have struck a familiar chord for many. When a group of businessmen were asked what five books they would choose if they were limited to five, *The Road Less Traveled* was a consistent choice. The author, M. Scott Peck, speaks of the ultimate goal of the human journey as the growth of the human spirit. The book begins, "Life is difficult. Once one accepts this fact, life becomes easier."

For many adults, successfully raising their children is their most meaningful challenge. For others, as described in recent books such as *Healthy Pleasures,* being involved in your community provides meaning and is actually *beneficial* to your health. In fact, studies of our longest-surviving citizens show that typically they have been actively involved with others throughout their lives. The ultimate measure of our lives may well be the degree to which we've been able to connect with others in our lifetime. And if you're lucky, along the way, you find your soul.

Recommendation

Find a philosophy, religion, or purpose in life larger than yourself in order to expand the meaning of your life.

Favorite Readings

The Road Less Traveled, by M. Scott Peck, M.D. New York: Simon & Schuster, 1978, 318 pgs.

Man's Search for Meaning, by Viktor Frankl, M.D. New York: Washington Square Press, 1984, 223 pgs.

When All You've Ever Wanted Isn't Enough, by Harold Kushner. New York: Pocket Books, 1986, 190 pgs.

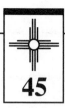

45

TAKE ONE STEP AT A TIME

Beware of being overly zealous! The greatest pitfall in making
behavior changes is trying to do too much at once. The result can be
injuries, discouragement (from not meeting goals that may have been
unrealistic to begin with), and resignation.

How to Use This Book

Pick one, two, or three (no more than three) chapters in this book on
which you'd like to focus. Or select a part of a chapter (perhaps the
chapter on stretching, but do three stretches in the morning instead of
six or ten). Write down which health areas you'd like to focus on:

1. _____
2. _____
3. _____

Ask yourself some questions about each change. What would you
call "success" in meeting that goal?

1. _____
2. _____
3. _____

What would you call "partial success"?

1. _____
2. _____
3. _____

What would be your first step toward meeting that goal?

1. _____
2. _____
3. _____

What is the single greatest cause for failure in attempting behavior changes?

When can you realistically expect to reach that first step?

1. _____
2. _____
3. _____

The next step?

1. _____
2. _____
3. _____

The last step?

1. _____
2. _____
3. _____

Choose times that you think are realistic for you, and write these times or dates down. Then write them in your appointment book or on a calendar. Some goals may be very short term, some may be seasonal or quarterly, and some may be annual.

Check in after a day, a week, and a month to see how you are doing. Every time you reach any step toward one of your goals, acknowledge yourself! If you slow down or think you have failed, *just start again.* When you see that one of your goals has become part of your life, you can pick a new one to work on if you choose. Be easy on yourself. Go slowly. And good luck.

Favorite Reading

Pathways: A Success Guide for a Healthy Life, Donald Kemper, M.P.H., Jim Giuffre, M.P.H., and Gene Drabinsky, R.N. Boise, ID: Healthwise, 1985, 145 pgs. Using the pathways compass in Chapter One is particularly helpful.

Answer:
Attempting to change too much at once

SUBJECT INDEX

WHO WANTS TO BE YOUNG & HEALTHY?

Everybody talks about the cost of health care.   So what are you going to do about it? Here's a suggestion: Give your friends and family copies of *Smart Ways to Stay Young & Healthy*. The practical suggestions in this book could add healthy years to their lives and save them thousands of dollars. The price is a bargain at $5.95. Order two copies or more and get generous discounts! You can even have a special premium edition printed to your specifications for your company or organization.

DISCOUNT & UPS SHIPPING SCHEDULE*

1 copy ....retail price, $5.95 per copy + $3 UPS per order

2 to 5 copies ....15% discount, $5.05 per copy + $3 UPS per order

6 to 25 copies ....25% discount, $4.47 per copy + $5 UPS per order

26 to 50 copies ....40% discount, $3.57 per copy + $8 UPS per order

51 to 100 copies ....50% discount, $2.98 per copy + $12 UPS per order

Over 100 copies ....call for special discounts

*terms & prices subject to change without notice

ORDER FORM : *SMART WAYS TO STAY YOUNG & HEALTHY*

_____ Quantity of books ordered

_____ x Price per copy (see discount   schedule)

_____ = Amount due for books

_____ x 8.25% sales tax (California residents only)

_____ + UPSshipping fee (USA only; see discount   schedule)

_____ = Total Amount Due

____ Check enclosed   Charge my __visa __ MC exp date ___ / ___/___

card # _____ / _____ / _____ / _____

Name _____

Address _____

City _____ State _____ Zip _____

Telephone # (_____) _____ - _____

For more information, or to place an order by phone call (510) 548-2124

or fill out the order form above and mail to

RONIN PUBLISHING Box 1035 Berkeley CA 94701

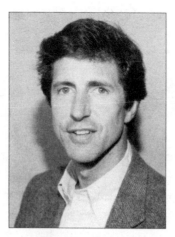

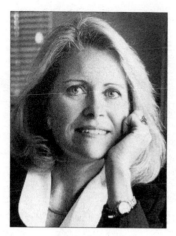

Bradley Gascoigne, M.D.

Julie Irwin

Dr. Bradley Gascoigne surveyed physicians to determine if they actually practice what they preach. He found that, while there are exceptions, good doctors usually take care of their own health. Thus, he found that a smart way of evaluating doctors is to consider how they take care of themselves.

Dr. Gascoigne is a staff physician with the Kaiser Permanente Medical Care Group of Northern California. He is Chairman of Kaiser Permanente Martinez Hospital's Patient and Health Education Committee, serves on Physician Well-Being and Employee Health Promotion committees in the San Francisco Bay Area and gives workshops on the importance of hobbies in peoples' lives. He was educated at University School in Cleveland, Ohio, Yale University, and University of Cincinnati Medical School. His internship was at San Francisco General Hospital, and his residency at University of New Mexico Medical Center. After working in the Public Health Service in Hyden, Kentucky, he was attending physician in the Emergency Department at Oakland Children's Hospital. Dr. Gascoigne lives in Oakland, California, and his own hobbies include jogging, flower arranging, and collecting old *New Yorker Magazine* covers.

Julie Irwin is an insurance industry expert promoting innovative changes and proposing cost saving ideas for medical and life insurance. She has worked in New Orleans City Government, and is a partner in Bryan Wagner Insurance, a company specializing in benefits for hospital employees. Julie serves on the Board of Governors for Tulane Medical Center and has served as a special consultant to Fortune 500 Hospital chains. She is active on a US Congressional Hospital Advisory Committee, the New Orleans Association of Life Underwriters, and a qualifying member of the Million Dollar Roundtable insurance group.

Julie Irwin is a graduate of Smith College. She lives in New Orleans with her husband Jim Irwin, an attorney, and her sons Jimmy and Chris. Her hobbies include horseback riding, hiking, skiing, jogging and gardening. Julie's work on this book is partially inspired by the words of Harold Kushner, "The Talmud says there are three things one should do in the course of one's life: have a child, plant a tree, and write a book."